OUTCOME OF THE
CRITICALLY ILL

MEDICINE, SURGERY AND TRAUMA

OUTCOME OF THE
CRITICALLY ILL

MEDICINE, SURGERY AND TRAUMA

Rade B. Vukmir, MD, JD
Director of Emergency Services,
NorthWest Medical Center,
Franklin, PA, USA

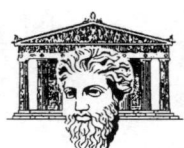

The Parthenon Publishing Group
International Publishers in Medicine, Science & Technology

NEW YORK   LONDON

Published in the USA by
The Parthenon Publishing Group Inc.
One Blue Hill Plaza
PO Box 1564, Pearl River
New York 10965, USA

Published in the UK and Europe by
The Parthenon Publishing Group Limited
Casterton Hall, Carnforth
Lancs., LA6 2LA, UK

Library of Congress Cataloging-in-Publication Data
Vukmir, Rade B.
  Outcome of the critically ill : medicine, surgery, and trauma / by Rade B. Vukmir.
    p. ; cm.
  Includes bibliographical references and index.
  ISBN 1-85070-903-3 (alk. paper)
  1. Critical care medicine--Handbooks, manuals, etc. 2. Surgical intensive care--
Handbooks, manuals, etc. 3. Outcome assessment (Medicinal care)--Handbooks,
manuals, etc. I. Title.
  [DNLM: 1. Critical Illness--Handbooks. 2. Treatment Outcome--Handbooks.
3. Hospital Mortality--Handbooks. 4. Intensive Care--methods--Handbooks.
WX 39 V989o 2000]
  RC86.7. V85 2000
  616'.028--dc21

                                                                    00-025525

British Library Cataloguing in Publication Data
Vukmir, Rade B.
  Outcome of the critically ill : medicine, surgery and trauma
  1. Critical care medicine
  I. Title
  616'.028

ISBN 1-85070-903-3

Typeset by Speedlith Photo Litho Ltd, Manchester, UK
Printed by J.W. Arrowsmith Ltd, Bristol, UK

Contents

Contents

Preface

It is impossible in this day and age to compose a book whose content is all things to all audiences. We have regressed towards specialization, subspecialization and 'micro-areas' of excellence. The intent of this compilation is to provide a comprehensive yet diverse international framework incorporating worldwide literature on outcome in the critically ill. This can help us to understand some of the intricacies of critical care medicine.

The intended audience includes those who have recently been exposed to the discipline or are in training, including medical students, residents and fellows. This group may benefit from the organ system-based analysis, which provides a framework for understanding complex critical care issues and dilemmas. In addition, the casual practitioner who does not routinely care for critically ill patients will find that the organ system framework allows informal prognostication based on individual organ system function or dysfunction.

Lastly, the expert critical care practitioner may benefit from the multidisciplinary nature of the information presented, which stresses medical, surgical, and anesthetic approaches to disease analysis. Likewise, the inclusion of rigorous programmed prognostication methods and scoring systems allows a better understanding and comparison of these individual outcome models.

The goal of this work was to provide a survey assessment of prognostication and prediction of clinical outcome in the critically ill. The design was orchestrated along three individual 'templates of understanding'. The first of these is the medical model, where typical issues encountered in a medical intensive care unit based on acute and subacute disease progression are presented. Specific studies and experimental models that predict clinically relevant outcome based on the involvement of a particular organ system are examined and compared. In addition, the cursory examination of cell-mediated cytokine

ix

response is also correlated with patient survival, morbidity, and mortality. Prognostication models that deal specifically with the care of the critically ill afflicted with medical conditions such as cardiac, respiratory or renal failure are examined and correlated to outcome.

Within the second 'template', anesthesia and surgical intensive care are explored in Section Two, which presents the surgical critical care model featuring pre-operative risk assessment in anesthesia, as well as care provided in the peri-operative phase of recovery. Conditions examined include those primary surgical problems resulting in significant illness such as intra-abdominal catastrophe, as well as multisystem organ involvement secondary to the rigors of surgery itself. An overall survey encompassing all aspects of general surgery, cardiovascular, transplant medicine, as well as the surgical sub-specialties such as plastic surgery and urology, are also included.

A significant proportion of critical care resources is directed towards the care of patients suffering multisystem trauma, and those with significant head injury. Probably no other disease array presents such a catastrophic loss of productive life capacity (in the case of acute traumatic injury) while yet resulting in such poor functional outcome (as can be associated with some catastrophic head injury). This third section allows us to examine and compare the program scoring systems specifically directed towards trauma management, as well as functional outcome predictors often associated with head and neurosurgical injury.

Hopefully, the reader will assimilate the information at hand and develop a careful, comprehensive strategy to care for the critically ill, analyzing all aspects of the disease process to maximize sensitivity by minimizing errors of omission. Later, this outline should be refined by the expert practitioner to increase diagnostic and therapeutic specificity, minimizing errors of commission. Ideally, this should allow us to provide the most benefit possible to patients and families so that realistic probability estimates may be presented, avoiding areas where the futility of patient care is overt.

Lastly, I have included specific sections addressing the cost and efficiency of care models, as well as the ethics of providing critical care to this patient population. I hope that I have emphasized a preventative aspect of critical care: that is, early intervention and avoidance of emergency intervention with its attendant risks and benefits is maximally beneficial. Ideally, careful planning and understanding of disease pathophysiology and patient monitoring will allow us to avoid both disease progression and iatrogenic complications.

My sincere appreciation goes to Christine Henderson for her tireless devotion to achieving this manuscript's endpoint.

This book is dedicated to my mother, Leni B. Vukmir, to whom I am indebted for providing the guidance to navigate through my various educational challenges.

R. B. Vukmir, MD, JD

1
Outcome of medical intensive care

INTRODUCTION

An early treatise on the development of the medical intensive care unit (MICU) was written by Callahan and colleagues in 1967 at St Mary's Hospital in Rochester, Minnesota, USA[1]. They suggested a 60% proportion of cardiovascular diagnosis, and meant to provide care to those 'critically but not hopelessly ill' with 'cardiac-mechanism failure'.

They also reported results of the care of 1000 patients admitted between 1964 and 1966[2]. The most common admission diagnosis was myocardial infarction (20%); 53% of patients were admitted from the emergency department with a mortality rate of 4.7% for cardiac and 10.7% for non-cardiac patients. Callahan and colleagues felt that care of both ICU patients and non-ICU patients was improved, as the care provided to the most ill patients did not deplete resources on the medical ward.

A report of the inaugural Norwegian ICU system at Ulleval Hospital in the University of Oslo described 30–36 ICU beds serving 300 medical beds, i.e. a 10% ratio of ICU/ward beds[3]. During the first year, 1801 patients were evaluated. The majority of these were treated for cardiac disease: 34% acute myocardial infarction (AMI), 33% general cardiac, 10% intoxications, 6% respiratory failure and 6% of admissions with gastrointestinal hemorrhage[3]. The mortality rate of the AMI patients was 24%, with circulatory arrest occurring in 192 (82% mortality), cardiogenic shock in 21% (76% mortality) and pulmonary edema in 35% (77% mortality); arrhythmia was diagnosed in 55% of AMI patients, with pacemaker insertion required in 10%.

Mortality in the tertiary-care referral and teaching centers is often more significant, compared to community centers, owing to patient selection bias. Spagnolo and associates reported a 47% mortality rate in a group of 213 tertiary-care patients with a wide age spectrum, including below age 20 years (0.5%), 20–24 years (3.8%), 30–39 years (5.6%),

40–49 years (24%), 50–59 years (30%), 60–69 years (17%), 70–79 years (15%) and 80 – 89 years (2.8% of the population)[4]. They noted the highest mortality in AMI patients (90%) and the lowest in those with asthma (0%), indicating a slight sample bias. An analysis by Thibault and co-workers of 2693 MICU patients at the Massachusetts General Hospital in Boston found a similar mortality rate of 58% during the study course[5].

The mortality pattern of a small (six-bed) MICU in a busy general hospital in Singapore reported 26% ICU and 42% hospital mortality rates[6]. This mortality appeared to be strongly associated with cardiac arrest, respirator support, duration of ICU stay, infection and immuno-compromised state. An additional factor appeared to be a lack of formal patient selection, entry criteria and dedicated critical care specialists.

The mortality of medical intensive care patients has been summarized in Table 1[2-7]; illustrating wide variance in outcome based on the patient population admitted.

Table 1 Medical intensive care mortality. Data from references 2–7, 108, 168, 192 and 204

Authors	Year	Hospital	Patients (n)	Mortality (%)	Cumulative incidence (per 1000)
Callahan et al.[2]	1967	St. Mary's, MN, USA	1000	7	0.007
Skjaeggestad et al.[3]	1970	Ulleval, Oslo, Norway	1801	10	0.099
Spagnolo et al.[4]	1973	Massachusetts General, MA, USA	213	47	0.470
Thibault et al.[5]	1980	Massachusetts General, MA, USA	2693	58	0.580
Chassin et al.[204]	1982		489	14	0.139
Tran et al.[168]	1990	Free University, Amsterdam, The Netherlands	487	27	0.270
Eng et al.[6]	1992	Singapore		26	
Fok et al.[192]	1992	Singapore General, Singapore	162	37	0.376
Lee et al.[108]	1993	National University, Singapore	131	37	0.370
Total			6976	31.8	0.306

DESIGN

In 1967 Staples reported the rapid development and expansion of the intensive care concept as it applied to nursing specialty development[7]. The article described unit design with a 'centralized station' and crash cart availability, as well as individual patient units monitoring nursing assignment with a team-oriented approach.

Skjaeggestad and colleagues felt that the Ulleval MICU was valuable[3], providing the advantages of:

(1) Effective and continuous 'round the clock' observation;

(2) Trained medical staff continuously available to utilize specialized equipment for immediate treatment; and

(3) Considerably improved opportunity to gain experience in the treatment of the critically ill patient.

Clark and associates reported the utility of the general-medical ICU in treating 60% of cardiac patients to be more related to a high staff/patient ratio than to the heavy capital spending on patient monitoring equipment, although the latter could be useful and sometimes vital[8].

Collins and co-workers, in a companion report on the Guy's Hospital experience in London, stressed the importance of simplicity in design, as each additional piece of monitoring equipment not only requires capital expenditure, but also increases demands on the nursing staff who are required to monitor cardiac, pressure and respiratory information[9].

Management

The question soon arose of what type of physician could best care for the patients. Clark and colleagues, from their experience at Guy's Hospital in 1971, suggested that, as the problems of critical care became more complex, no single doctor was likely to be competent enough to provide all ICU services, as there was no intensive care equivalent of the general physician[8].

Mushin and Lunn explored the inadequacies of the system in 1969, with the contention that 'anesthesiologists may not be best suited to care for myocardial infarction and cardiologists are ill-advised to pontificate on hemodialysis, and the all-purpose intensivist must remain a will-o'-the-wisp with their availability not then achievable'[10].

During early ICU development, it was suggested that the intensive care system was likely to function best using a divisional specialist system of critical care, matching particular specialty expertise with the disease process.

In the past, the focus has been on survival, but the target must now be legitimate functional recovery end-point markers. The mixed ICU population of 2693 patients evaluated by Thibault and co-workers[5] was responsible for a significant proportion of total hospital charges (37%), mortality (58%) occurring predominantly in the aged, chronically ill who received active medical intervention. However, the actual intensive care mortality rate reported was half of that occurring on the general medical ward.

The institution of a dedicated critical care service can be associated with improved outcome, as studied in 212 MICU patients by Reynolds and colleagues[11], with a decrease in mortality from 74% to 54% reported. This population was matched for significant injury severity (Acute Physiology and Chronic Health Evaluation, APACHE score 28–29) with another population not cared for by a critical care service, and received more aggressive intravascular monitoring including both arterial (73% vs 24%) and pulmonary artery (64% vs 48%) catheterization.

Family practice ICU admissions were analyzed in 1983, and it was found that 38% of residency faculties had admission privileges in university teaching hospitals, with a minority requiring mandatory referral to an ICU specialist[12]. However, a study by Hainer and Lawler[13] of 523 medical and coronary care cases, comparing patients of family practitioners and internal medical physicians, suggested no difference in mortality rate (36% vs. 38%), charges ($US 4318 vs. $US 5155) or number of referrals (0.8 vs. 0.7). This specific ICU patient population, however, was only of minor illness severity according to the APACHE II scoring criteria; this may have contributed to the outcome.

Carson and associates evaluated the effect of an organizational change on ICU operation, in the transition from 'open' to 'closed' treatment formats for 245 patients[14]. Patients in the 'closed' ICU group cared for by dedicated ICU practitioners had more severe illness in terms of APACHE II score (15.4–20.6), but a lower ratio of observed (relative risk 0.78, 31–40%) to predicted (relative risk 0.90, 23–25%)

mortality. The nurses subjectively (41% vs. 7%) felt more comfortable with physician clinical judgement, although there was no difference in length of stay (3.7 days vs. 3.9 days) or use of radiology, laboratory and pharmacy resources for the patients of dedicated critical care practitioners.

SPECIAL RISK GROUPS

The consideration of medical conditions and associated mortality results in the finding that analysis of specific diseases and organ systems may enhance prognostic ability (Table 2).

Information about mortality can be found by review of MICU or coronary care unit autopsy data. Campion and associates reported the results of 1080 consecutive deaths with an overall autopsy rate of 36%[15]. The autopsy rate declined sharply with age, from 60% for those aged 16–34 years to 23% for those aged over 85 years. The most common diagnoses defined by the examination were aortic aneurysm (70%), hepatic failure (52%), heart rhythm disturbance (48%), pulmonary embolism (45%) and sepsis (41%). Patients having undergone major procedures had a higher autopsy rate (38% vs. 29%), as a direct result of the investigation of post-procedural complications.

AIDS

The presence of acquired immunodeficiency syndrome (AIDS) is a significant predictor of morbidity and mortality in the MICU patient. Rodgers and colleagues evaluated 216 MICU admissions of AIDS patients. Twenty-three percent of these had been admitted for life-sustaining therapy, which was required for respiratory failure caused predominantly by *Pneumocystis carinii* pneumonia in 36 of the 50 patients[16]. The 3-month mortality rate of this group was 74%; however, 25 needlestick injuries and exposure to 56 mucosal splashes resulted in not a single seroconversion in medical personnel.

Survival rates were predicted from the time of initial hospital admission for respiratory failure to be 47% immediate-hospital and 37% 1-year survival, from Friedman and colleagues' series of 73 AIDS patients[17]. Therefore, the presence of respiratory failure does not necessarily signify the terminal phase of human immunodeficiency

Table 2 Medical conditions and associated mortality. Data from references 4, 16–18, 20, 24–26, 30, 54, 55, 57, 59, 60, 64, 68, 84, 88, 89–91, 94–96, 98, 99, 107–109, 126, 130, 139, 140 and 147

| | Mortality (%) | | |
| | | Discharge | |
Disease	*Hospital*	*3 months*	*1 year*
AIDS	53		63
Geriatric (>75 years) complications	67		44
Cardiac arrest	89–91		
Malignancy	90		
Cardiac			
AMI	13		16
AMI with complications	90		
congestive heart failure	23		
hypertension	10		
syncope			19
Pulmonary			
ARF	78		
chronic illness	71–93		
mechanical ventilation	33–44	38	46–77
asthma	0–11		
ARDS	50–80		
Infectious disease	47–62		
septicemia	91		
polymicrobial	67–87		
Gastrointestinal			
pancreatitis	33		
UGIB	21–64		
hemorrhage	62		
Hepatic	64		
cirrhosis	83		
cirrhosis with hemorrhage	77		
Renal	57–63		
Immunology			
anergy	32		
Hematology			
malignancy	21–75%		
bone marrow transplant	22–33%		
untreated	87%		
Oncology	10%		

Table 2   Continued

6

Table 2 *Continued*

Disease	Hospital	Mortality (%) Discharge 3 months	1 year
Endocrine			
diabetes mellitus with complications	27		
hypocalcemia	44		
Rheumatology	33	42	
Neurology			
cerebrovascular accident	60–75		
Toxicology	5–7		
propoxyphene	8		
Psychiatry			
neuroleptic malignancy syndrome	20		

AMI, acute myocardial infarction; ARF, acute respiratory failure; ARDS, adult respiratory distress syndrome; UGIB, upper gastrointestinal bleeding

virus (HIV) infection, making those with AIDS appropriate candidates for life-supporting therapy when clear guidelines have been established.

The presence of concurrent bacterial infection with bacteremia in 29 patients with AIDS was at a level of 10%, which was less than the 17% rate found in spinal-cord injury control patients[18]. Pulmonary infection did not occur more commonly in those who were intubated, nor did it affect the incidence of survival in those with respiratory failure. Thus, intubation should not be withheld owing to concerns about bacterial superinfection in those who have the clinical syndrome of AIDS.

The predictive ability of the APACHE II scoring system has been applied to HIV-positive patients by Brown and Crede, who found a significant underestimation of actual mortality rate: 35% predicted vs. 44% observed[19]. Specifically, the mortality risk was predicted accurately for those with a total lymphocyte count of $\geq$ 201 cells/mm^3 (33%), but mortality was underestimated (44% vs. 61%) in those with a total lymphocyte count of < 200 cells/mm^3, especially in those with pneumonia or sepsis (50% vs. 88%).

Geriatrics

The impact of age on ICU admission practices was examined in 599 ICU and 290 ward patients categorized into under 55 years, 55–64 years, 65–74 years and 75 years and over age groups[20]. Older patients (more than 65 years) comprised 48% of the MICU sample, while 21% of those under 55 years had no prior chronic illness compared to less than 8% of older patients. Although hospital survival declines with age from 85 to 70%, survival adjusted for chronic health conditions was equivalent. Therefore, age had no appreciable impact on survival in this evaluation.

Campion and associates examined 2693 medical intensive and coronary care unit admissions, noting that older patients were more likely to receive major life support interventions such as mechanical ventilation, but were less likely to survive[21]. Major interventions were used in 32% of those aged 75 years or older, 26% of those aged 65–74 years and 22% of those aged 55–64 years, associated with mortality rates of 16%, 14% and 8%, respectively and a 1-year mortality rate of 44% for those older than 75 years. Nonetheless, elderly patients had neither a longer hospital stay nor greater hospital charges.

Older patients have sometimes been excluded from ICUs because of the perception that they will benefit less than younger patients. Wu and co-workers performed a retrospective examination of 130 'old' (above 75 years) and 135 'moderately aged' (55–65 years) patients, controlling for severity of illness[22]. The older group was afflicted with increased incidence of chronic obstructive pulmonary disease, longer hospital stay (39 days vs. 37 days) and greater mortality (51% vs. 39%). However, when logistic regression was used to adjust for APACHE II score modified to exclude age, the presence of a privately attending physician, primary admission diagnosis or presence of cancer, older patients did not have a significantly greater risk of dying (adjusted relative risk 1.05, 95% confidence interval 0.97–1.12).

The nursing-home patient is often relegated to a less aggressive treatment pathway implicitly. Goldstein and colleagues evaluated 1256 patients, comparing those residing in a nursing home ($n = 67$), those receiving home care ($n = 240$) and all other geriatric (above 65 years) patients, comprising 37% of total ICU admissions[23]. Nursing-home patients were most likely to be admitted with cardiopulmonary arrest, infection and gastrointestinal bleeding, as opposed to acute ischemic heart disease for younger patients. Although the major interventions, i.e. intubation and mechanical ventilation were more frequent in nursing-home patients, the total hospital charges differed little among groups.

The in-hospital mortality rate for the nursing-home group (28%) was significantly higher than those for the home-care group (7%) and older patients (7%). Hence, cumulative mortality for the nursing-home group reached 66% by 8 months, compared to 32% for the home-care and 26% for the normal geriatric population.

Complications

The nature of iatrogenic complications is complex and potentially impacts on ICU outcome. Rubins and Moskowitz evaluated 295 patients admitted to the MICU and found that 42 (14%) of them experienced one or more complications during their ICU stay, resulting in a significant increase in mortality, compared to those experiencing no complications (67% vs. 27%)[24]. Those patients who experienced complications tended to be older (64 years vs. 59 years), be more acutely ill (acute physiology score 18 vs. 12) and have a longer ICU length of stay (12 days vs. 3 days). ICU complications are not rare, therefore, and may independently contribute to hospital mortality.

CARDIOPULMONARY ARREST

Significant advantage would be achieved if premonitory signs predictive of cardiac arrest could be elicited by health-care personnel prior to the event itself. Franklin and Mathew evaluated 150 cardiac-arrest patients on the medical ward, with an incidence of 7.0/1000 patients and a hospital mortality rate of 91%[25]. In 99 (66%) cases, there was documented evidence of clinical deterioration in the patients' condition within 6 h of cardiac arrest. Issues of significance include:

(1) Failure of the nurse to notify a physician of deterioration in the patient's mental status;

(2) Failure of the physician to obtain or interpret an arterial blood gas measurement in the setting of respiratory distress;

(3) Failure of the ICU triage physician to stabilize the patient's condition before ICU transfer.

In addition, patients who had suffered previous cardiac arrest (14.7/1000) were more likely to suffer cardiac arrest than other patients (6.8/1000).

Therefore, it is desirable to monitor changes in mental status indicative of impending arrest, preventing deterioration with early intervention, especially in those who have suffered a previous cardiac arrest.

The issue of successful resuscitation in critical care units assumes importance because patients often have multisystem disorders that may be responsible for poor outcome post-cardiopulmonary resuscitation. Peterson and associates reviewed the records of 114 MICU patients with a 70% mortality rate; 18% were successfully resuscitated but died prior to discharge, while 11% of patients survived to discharge[26]. The pre-arrest conditions of hypotension, sepsis and APACHE II acute physiology score elevation, and the arrest conditions of duration of resuscitation effort, are independently associated with poor outcome post-cardiopulmonary resuscitation. However, cardiopulmonary resuscitation can be successful in ICU patients, and both pre-arrest and arrest variables can be predictive of outcome.

CARDIAC

Syncope is often a patient-presenting complaint that is historically addressed with admission to a monitored setting. Silverstein and associates reviewed 108 patients admitted to the MICU, where, in 36% of syncope cases a cardiac cause was defined, 17% were due to non-cardiovascular disease and 47% were of unknown etiology[27]. The 1-year mortality rate was 19% in the cardiovascular group, 6% in the non-cardiovascular group and 6% for the idiopathic cases, the last figure comparable to the rate for the normal population.

Identifying patients at low risk for complications of myocardial events may encourage decreased admissions and earlier discharge from the unit. Risk stratification of 360 patients with uncomplicated chest pain found 168 (47%) without major complications, elevation of creatine phosphokinase (CPK) levels or electrocardiographic evidence of transmural infarction[28]. This 'low-risk' group subsequently met criteria for infarct in 3% of cases, with 2% having late ICU complications, but no patients succumbed. The evidence suggested that identification of low-risk patients could reduce total bed days by 55%.

Predictive factors in medical patients include the presence of arrhythmia, occurring as a marker of cardiac disease, which can have adverse prognostic significance. Gulsvik and colleagues evaluated 451 patients with severe pulmonary disease; where 39% developed a major cardiac arrhythmia during their ICU stay which was associated with increased mortality, compared to those patients with pulmonary disease who did not develop arrhythmia (31% vs. 8%)[29]. However, it was difficult to separate the adverse outcome of cardiac disease from the effects of the pulmonary disease alone.

The most common reason for monitored admission is the suspicion of ischemia. Fernandes and co-workers described their experience of 55 patients with the diagnosis of unstable angina admitted to the MICU, where 95% had primary angina and 5% had post-infarction angina[30]. Most patients went on to require revascularization, 62% by percutaneous transluminal coronary angioplasty (PCTA) and 13% by coronary artery bypass graft (CABG), and all patients survived.

The usefulness of the APACHE II scoring system has been explored to aid in prognostication of in-hospital mortality in acute myocardial infarction. Ludwigs and Hulting reported the experience of 1714 patients with mean age 72 ± 10 years, ICU mortality rate of 13%, total hospital mortality of 16% and mean APACHE II score of 11.6 ± 6.5[31]. There was good correlation between observed and predicted scores while, in the more severely affected (APACHE II 20–24), the APACHE II system underestimated mortality in those who stayed less than 8 h in the MICU. Therefore, the APACHE II system was a reasonable predictor for cardiac patients except for the most severely affected.

Surgical intervention may improve survival rates, and the quality of life of those who have undergone urgent cardiac transplantation is excellent; this is a viable option for end-stage cardiac disease. Mulcahy and colleagues evaluated 18 patients who required aggressive chemical and mechanical support in the ICU to find that 95% survived 5 years, with 61% not restricted in the activities of daily living and 55% working full-time[32].

MONITORING

Early studies by Wiener and Weil in 1977 reported on the specifics of ICU computer-based monitoring systems, stressing the need for monitoring of basic vital signs, core temperature and cardiac output, narrative data entry, process control and data retrieval[33]. They suggested automated fluid challenge, mechanical ventilation alternations and fluid therapy to increase ICU efficiency, an idea being proposed today.

Computer-assisted monitoring systems have been utilized to assist in arrhythmia detection. Alcover and colleagues described a computer-assisted monitoring system that compared algorithmic analysis with the interpretation of critical-care physicians[34]. The incidence of false-positive diagnosis or computer system errors ranged from 10 in 1000 beats for critically ill patients on volume ventilation, those with uncomplicated myocardial infarction and those undergoing telemetry monitoring to 20 in 1000 for pacemaker-dependent patients. Movement artifact accounted for 55.3% of false-positive diagnoses, and the most frequent true positive was pacemaker malfunction, diagnosed with 94% accuracy.

A more mundane aspect of ICU care is the need to monitor urine output. Jain and associates compared 135 MICU and 67 medical floor patients in terms of the prevalence of unjustified catheter placement and monitoring[35]. The initial indication for the placement of a urinary catheter was unjustified in 21% of 202 patients, while continued use was unjustified in 47% of the 912 patient-days. In the MICU, 64% of the total unjustified patient-days of catheter placement were maintained to 'monitor urine output'. Urinary incontinence was the major cause of both unjustified initial (52%) and continued (56%) use of catheters in floor patients, while only 5% were maintained for continuous bladder irrigation. Therefore, a careful, conservative catheterization plan will avoid later ICU morbidity and mortality, with minimal use of long-term indwelling catheterization for incontinence, or marginal 'fluid monitoring' considerations.

Coincidentally, Roos and colleagues, in an evaluation of fluid assessment technology, found no reliable relationship between calculated weight changes using fluid balances corrected for insensible losses and observed weight changes[36]. They concluded that absolute weight measurements are indispensable.

Laboratories often collect more blood than is needed for specific tests and measurements. Dale and Pruett evaluated 113 MICU patients during a 1-week period of blood draws to find sampling often 45 (range 2–102) fold overestimation of the volume of blood required[37]. Thus, minimizing the number and volume of blood draws will avoid iatrogenic anemia, infection and an increase in direct and indirect costs.

Another area of particular concern in the setting of cost-conscious practice is that of arterial blood gas monitoring. Venkatesh and co-workers reported the results of a trial of a continuous intra-arterial blood gas monitor[38]. They defined an overall bias ± precision value of 0.01 ± 0.06 for pH, 1.4 ± 4.8 torr (0.2 ± 0.7 kPa) for pCO_2 and 2.8 ± 25.6 torr (0.4 ± 3.4 kPa) for pO_2, and a mean *in vivo* response time of 78, 143 and 70 s, respectively. This device was able continuously to track arterial blood gas parameters without the need for intermittent sampling.

Zimmerman and Dellinger performed a similar small study of five patients each with an indwelling fiberoptic sensor placed through a 20-gauge arterial catheter[39]. The comparison of sensor with blood gas analyzer values reported bias and precision values of -0.021 and 0.037 for arterial pH, 1.74 and 6.06 torr (0.23 and 0.81 kPa) for $paCO_2$ and -5.89 and 13.19 torr (-0.79 and 1.76 kPa) for paO_2. The performance of this sensor was adequate in reliably approximating the arterial pH, paO_2 and $paCO_2$ values without patient morbidity.

An area of recent development is the use of devices and techniques to minimize iatrogenic blood loss. Silver and co-workers reported their experience with a blood loss conservation system for arterial sampling in 31 patients in a prospective cross-over design[40]. The mean total volume of blood sampled over a 7-day period for testing was 258 ml, and those patients in whom the conventional system, which had to have the 'line cleared', was used lost an additional 157 ml of blood, compared to those in whom the blood conserving system was used. These results assume significance when compared with the volume of packed red blood cells for transfusion of 450 ml.

In a similar evaluation, Peruzzi and colleagues followed 100 MICU patients and found less blood drawn and discarded in the blood conservation group both from arterial catheters (95.7ml vs. 96.4 ml) and in total (19.4 ml vs. 103.5 ml), as well as an increase in hemoglobin levels by 1.2 ± 2.2 g/dl[41]. However, statistical significance in decreased blood sampling was not reached until 9 days into the study, mandating a cost–benefit analysis of salvage systems.

Pulmonary artery catheter

The use of the pulmonary artery catheter was first report in 1970 by Ganz and associates, using end-diastolic pressure to estimate preload and end-systolic volume to estimate contractility or afterload[42]. Myocardial performance was measured as cardiac output calculated by the thermodilution technique, where a fixed volume of injectate is used to predict flow by measurement of the change in temperature between two fixed points, cardiac output being equal to volume multiplied by temperature change over time (CO = $V \times T°/\text{time}$)[43].

The spontaneous variability of cardiac output over time in critically ill patients is acknowledged. Sasse and colleagues performed a real-time evaluation of thermodilution cardiac output variability, demonstrating an overall mean coefficient of variation of 5.8% at single point and 7.7% over time[44]. Further subgroup analysis defined the 'stable' group with a 6.4% coefficient of variation and the 'unstable' group with a 9.9% coefficient of variation over time, as well as variance in mechanical ventilation (6.4%) and spontaneous respiration (10.1%). Hence, assuming a baseline cardiac output of 10.0 l/min, the 'unstable' patient had a cardiac output varying in the range of 8.8–11.2 l/min.

Unger and colleagues evaluated 14 adult respiratory distress syndrome patients and defined four (29%) as having left-ventricular failure with pulmonary artery occulsion pressure of > 12 mmHg[45]. This early study suggested no clinical or laboratory parameters that could identify these patients prospectively, and appropriate therapeutic end-points were obtained in three of the four (75%) patients.

The inherent issues with the use of these and other sophisticated medical interventions include the accuracy of physician prediction of hemodynamic profiles, and whether a beneficial change in therapy and outcome is generated. Mimoz and associates evaluated 112 MICU patients where 38% of pulmonary artery catheters were placed in those with unresponsive shock syndromes. Following catheter placement, hemodynamic profiles were correctly predicted prospectively in only 56% and therapeutic changes occurred in 58% of patients, with 33% of these incurring fluid overload and 87% being hypovolemic[46]. There were complications in 9.8% of patients, including pneumothorax and arrhythmia, but only two required therapy. There was no overall change in outcome following catheter placement, except in the unresponsive shock patients, for whom the mortality rate was significantly improved (59% vs. 100%) in those with pulmonary artery catheter placement.

The potential impact of pulmonary artery catheter placement on short-term management decisions in the ICU was explored in 103 patients with indications for placement of refractory congestive heart failure, airspace disease, uncertain cardiac filling pressure or hypotension[47]. In over half of the patients (56%), management recommendations changed as a direct result of information obtained from the pulmonary artery catheter. These changes involved fluid therapy recommendations in 41, (40%), intravenous vasodilator use in 24, (23%), vasopressor use in 17 (16%) and isotropic agent use in 15 (15%). However, 18 (17%) patients experienced early or late complications, with major events limited to pneumothorax in one (0.9%) and bacterium in four (4%). Hence, benefits achieved by significant management alterations in the critically ill can offset the complication rate and, although no deaths were directly attributable to catheter insertion in the above study, the morbidity factors must nevertheless be considered.

An important consideration in the use of these devices relates to the complications of insertion and use. In a study by Plit and colleagues, the acute complication rate included 2.8% incidence of pneumothorax and 2.2% incidence of arteral puncture, there was a chronic complication rate of 3.6% for sepsis, and balloon dysfunction occurred in 6% of cases of vascular cannulation[48].

A well-publicized concern is the risk of complete heart block in those with left-bundle branch block. Morris and associates reported on 82 pulmonary artery catheterizations and found no new cases of complete heart block in those with old or indeterminate block, and only two (2%) cases of new block occurring over 24 h after placement[49]. Therefore, routine placement of a prophylactic temporary transvenous pacemaker is probably not warranted even in the MICU population.

Additional information gleaned from the use of the pulmonary artery catheter includes the benefit of oximetric monitoring. Fahey and co-workers evaluated oximetric monitoring of 86 critically ill patients over a range of mixed venous oxygen saturations from 24 to 85%, noting a correlation coefficient between *in vivo* SvO_2 and photometrically measured samples of 0.95[50]. The mean duration of usage in the MICU was 6.1 days, demonstrating a strong correlation (0.88) between oxygen delivery and SvO_2 in nine of 13 patients studied. Those patients for whom correlation was suboptimal were usually affected by sepsis.

Oxygen supply and demand relationships can be defined by both invasive (pulmonary artery catheterization) and non-invasive (expiratory gas analysis) methods. Kreymann and colleagues analyzed the oxygen consumption and metabolic rate by respired gas analysis to

15

define oxygen consumption (V_{O_2}), basal metabolic rate, oxygen delivery (D_{O_2}) and oxygen extraction ration (V_{O_2}/D_{O_2}) in sepsis in nine patients (Table 3)[51]. In sepsis syndrome, the oxygen consumption and basal metabolic rate were increased by 30% compared to normal values, but were markedly decreased compared to uncomplicated sepsis; the higher oxygen consumption found in uncomplicated sepsis was flow independent. During recovery from sepsis syndrome or septic shock, the basal metabolic rate increased to 61 ± 22%.

Hence, either direct assessment via expiratory gas analysis or indirect assessment via pulmonary artery thermodilution technology can help to track disease progression and recovery in sepsis.

The use of a combined catheter, featuring continuous oximetry and volume as well as pressure measurement, has an advantage over standard monitoring. The end-diastolic volume has been proved to be a more reliable means of estimating preload than pulmonary artery occlusion pressure in the critically ill population[52].

Finally, the tetrapolar impedance technique has been explored in 31 MICU patients by Roos and co-workers in a model where dehydrated subjects had resistances of > 700 Ω, while resistances of < 400 Ω were found in those who were edematous[53]. A 60% cut-off level for discriminate analysis found no false-positive predictions, suggesting a benefit of this non-invasive monitoring technique.

The most recent comprehensive evaluation of 5735 critically ill patients by the SUPPORT investigators correlated the use of right-heart catheterization in the first 24 h of ICU care with survival, length of stay, intensity of care and costs of care. Those patients who

Table 3 Oxygen consumption and metabolic rate in sepsis. Table adapted from reference 51

	Sepsis	*Sepsis syndrome*	*Septic shock*	*Significance*
Oxygen consumption V_{O_2} (ml/min/m²)	180 ± 19	156 ± 22	120 ± 27	$p < 0.001$
Resting metabolic rate (%)	55 ± 14	24 ± 12	2 ± 24	$p < 0.001$
Oxygen delivery D_{O_2} (ml/min/m²)	501 ± 116	515 ± 186	404 ± 96	
Oxygen extraction	0.36	0.30	0.29	

underwent catheterization had increased 30-day mortality rate, mean cost of hospital stay ($US 49 300 vs. $US 39 200) and length of stay (14.8 days vs. 13.0 days), compared to those who did not undergo catheterization. However, limitations of the study include its observational design, even after adjustment for treatment selection bias[54].

The obvious next step would be a randomized controlled trial of the pulmonary artery catheter to determine the cost/benefit ratio in the ICU population specifically.

PULMONARY

Perhaps the most significant proportion of critical care resources is devoted to the ICU management of primary or secondary respiratory failure. Primary causes of pulmonary insufficiency include pneumonia, asthma and chronic obstructive pulmonary disease exacerbation, while secondary causes include pulmonary edema, sepsis and neurological dysfunction.

Acute respiratory failure is a common occurrence, reported in 89 (6%) of the total and 332 (21%) of mechanically ventilated patients in a series of 1594 patients studied by Goeckenjan and colleagues[55]. Those with acute respiratory failure presented at a younger age, with female predominance and longer duration of ventilation resulting in a higher mortality (79% vs. 58%), compared to more chronically ill patients. Prognostic factors included underlying disease, additional organ dysfunction, severity of pulmonary gas exchange and advanced age. The most favourable outcomes were found in single organ system failure with change in arterial pO_2 of < 250 mmHg (33% mortality) and after hypovolemic shock, pancreatitis or postoperative pulmonary failure (65% mortality); the least favorable outcomes were found with septicemia, peritonitis, cirrhosis, esophageal varices or polytrauma with acute renal failure, with a mortality rate of over 80%.

Mechanical ventilation in the elderly was evaluated by Swinburne and colleagues in 1860 patients, comparing two groups, those older and those younger than 80 years of age[56]. They found that survival was slightly worsened (38% vs. 49%) in the elderly without premorbid illness, but was significantly worsened (7% vs. 29%) for those with pre-existing renal, hepatic or gastrointestinal disease with malnutrition or malignancy. Thus, in the very old, chronically ill patient where chances

17

for meaningful survival are small, support withdrawal was recommended. However, there was little change in survival based on age alone, so limitations to geriatric care may not be appropriate.

The Veterans' Affairs Cooperative Study examined predictors of outcome in 612 mechanically ventilated patients who demonstrated hospital survival of 56%, decreasing to a 1-year survival rate of 23%[57]. A patient subset for whom aggressive support provided little or no benefits included those over 70 years, demonstrating a 6% 1-year survival, hypoalbuminemia (2.0 mg/dl) in 4%, an APACHE II score of >35 in 2% and 10% survival at 1 year following cardipulmonary resuscitation.

Ludwigs and co-workers performed a large-scale evaluation of mechanical ventilation in the MICU, where 1008 (4%) of 24 899 patients required support[58]. The mean age of ventilation-treated patients was 53 ± 18 years, with an average duration of ventilation of 4.7 days. The MICU mortality rate was 33%, with hospital mortality of 38% and 2-year mortality of 46%. Cerebrovascular (75%) and malignant (79%) disease carried the highest mortality rates, while drug overdose carried the lowest mortality rate (2%). It was found to be helpful to define the prognosis by classification of disease syndromes based on system involvement.

Asthma

Acute asthma or related bronchospasm is unique in that the condition is often not reversed and may actually be worsened by intubation and mechanical ventilation. Braman and Kaemmerlen evaluated 80 patient episodes of status asthmaticus and found 50 (62.5%) with respiratory failure, i.e. $paco_2 > 50$ mmHg[59]. Mechanical ventilation was required in only half of the patients with severe acidosis and hypercapnia, and most patients improved rapidly, requiring only a short ICU stay, contrary to prior experience suggesting a high mortality.

Clinical characteristics of 38 patients with severe asthma found presentations of hypoxemia, hypercapnia (pco_2 54 mmHg) and decreased peak flow rates of 125.5 l/min[60]. Patients spent approximately 2.5 days in the MICU where 45% required mechanical ventilation, but all patients survived, indicating the utility of aggressive management.

Additional mortality data can be inferred from Lim's small study of 19 consecutive episodes of status asthmaticus admitted to the MICU, where 11 of 19 required mechanical ventilation with an 11% (2/19) mortality rate[61]. He reported that most patients had respiratory acidosis and, although this was not predictive of ventilation requirement, the peak inspiratory pressure was a valid index of underlying lung disease and was associated with the most serious complication – barotrauma.

Bartter and Pratter performed a meta-analysis of care provided by both 'experts' and 'generalists' in a general medical population presenting with life-threatening asthma[62]. The 'expert or specialist' based systems provided better medical outcome, at a lower cost, for this disease condition.

Pneumonia

Severe pneumonia can often require intensive monitoring and therapy. The experience of Dahmash and Chowdhury with 113 patients found culture-proven diagnosis in 80% of patients, with single organisms isolated in 69% of cases. The most frequent was *Pseudomonas aeruginosa* in 16% followed by *Streptococcus pneumoniae* (12%), *Staphylococcus aureus* (9%) and *Mycobacterium tuberculosis* in 8%[63]. The overall mortality was 17% higher in hospital-acquired pneumonia cases for those with serious underlying disease, abnormal mental status, diastolic blood pressure <60 mmHg, blood urea >7 mmol/l, abnormal liver function, albumin <3.0 g/l, mechanical ventilation and APACHE II score > 20. Preventing the onset or minimizing the severity of associated organ system failure in the setting of pulmonary infection may potentially improve outcome.

There were 74 cases of pneumonia admitted to the MICU in the series of Limthongkul and Charoenlap, with 46 (62%) community-, 26 (35%) hospital- and two (3%) combined-acquired infections[64]. The majority of patients had underlying pulmonary disease, and had been admitted with respiratory failure (85%), with mechanical ventilation requirement. The overall mortality rate was 63.5% owing to uncontrolled pneumonia in 38% and complications of mechanical ventilation in 26%. The duration of mechanical ventilation was 13.8 days, ICU stay was 13.2 days and hospital stay was 29 days. High-risk factors associated with non-survival were assisted ventilation, ventilation complications, shock and Gram-negative infection. However, those who required mechanical ventilation did so as a result of their underlying disease as much as the current infectious condition.

Adult respiratory distress syndrome

The adult respiratory distress syndrome (ARDS) has remained one of the most lethal complications in both medical and surgical ICUs, with mortality rates of 50–80%[65]. Risk factors include sepsis, direct pulmonary injury from aspiration, contusion and near-drowning. Pathophysiological mechanisms implicated include granulocyte aggregation with formation of oxygen free radicals as well as other mediators.

The occurrence of pulmonary barotrauma is often the initiating factor in ARDS development. Gammon and colleagues evaluated 139 mechanically ventilated patients to discover a 25% incidence of barotrauma, and 17% of these patients had mediastinal emphysema[66]. The presence of mediastinal emphysema was associated with a positive predictive value of 42% for pneumothorax, which occurred in ten of 24 patients. ARDS patients had the highest risk for barotrauma, followed by chronic obstructive pulmonary disease and pneumonia. Those patients had higher peak inspiratory pressure, positive end expiratory pressure, respiratory rate, tidal volume and minute ventilation exhibiting significantly elevated values resulting in a greater incidence of barotrauma and ARDS.

There are few controlled studies of ventilatory effectiveness, but a strategy to minimize FiO_2 by optimizing PEEP and decreasing barotrauma by controlled ventilation using sedation has been reported[65]. The use of pressure control ventilation, in which ventilation volume becomes the dependent variable, may serve to prevent barotrauma from causing further lung injury[67].

Impaired fibrinolysis may contribute to the development of ARDS, as a result of a pathological increase in endogenous plasminogen activator inhibitor-1 (PAI-1) that blunts normal fibrinolysis and unmasks an alternative fibrinolytic mechanism, such as elastase-induced fibrin degradation. Moalli and co-workers evaluated 71 MICU patients, and found ARDS patients to have significantly higher levels of PAI-1 as well as the acute lung injury markers, including factor VIII-related antigen (VIII:Ag) and α-1-protease inhibitor (α-1-PI)[68]. Certainly, further studies will need to be carried out to elucidate these relationships.

INFECTIOUS DISEASE

Early discussion of infectious disease complications centered on colonization and superinfection in ICU patients. A survey of infection in critically ill patients has been offered by Dahmash and colleagues, who reviewed their experience with 105 MICU patients[69]. The overall incidence of infection was 47%, acquired in the medical ward in the majority (48%), but also acquired in the community (27%) and in the MICU (25%). The most frequent infections by far were pneumonia and septicemia, accounting for 88% of the total; others were urinary tract (4.4%), gastrointestinal tract (5.0%) and skin and wound (2.5%) infections, with an overall study mortality rate of 42%.

Nosocomial infection

The transition from ICU colonist to nosocomial pathogen is often accompanied by worsened outcome. Craven and associates evaluated 526 MICU and 799 surgical ICU patients, with the rate of nosocomial infection being higher in the latter group (31% vs. 24%)[70]. The surgical ICU patients had more urinary tract infections, bacteria, wound infections and reviewed prior antibiotics, and more likely endotracheal tube, intravascular catheter and bladder catheter placement, while the MICU patients were more likely to be older, have higher acute physiology score, present with shock or coma and have a higher fatality rate (18%).

Colonization versus infection

A prospective epidemiological survey found that hand-washing samples revealed pathogenic bacteria in 31% of physicians, with 71 300 colony-forming units per hand, and in 17% of nurses, with 39 800 colony-forming units per hand. Airborne particle sampling was positive in 15% of cases, and 17% (9 of 53) of patients were found to be colonized with Gram-negative, *S. aureus* or *Candida* species[71]. The direct contact mode of transmission was confirmed as responsible for most iatrogenic transfer of organisms, as the airborne pathogens appeared not to have been implicated. Therefore, for the above species (but not mycobacteria), hand washing appeared to be more effective than ventilation system improvement.

Rose and Babcock studied 64 patients, comparing medical and surgical ICU populations, to document pharyngeal colonization in 22% and 39% and intestinal colonization with Gram-negative rods in

21

19% and 41%, respectively[72]. They concluded that the higher colonization rate in surgical patients was a result of indwelling catheters, while the prevalence in medical patients was a result of antibiotic use.

Specific pathogens

Another area of concern is the rapid development of resistant enterococci in the ICU. In a prospective study, the prevalence of ampicillin-resistant enterococci was 5.4% and that of vancomycin-resistant enterococci was 1.12%[73]. Prior hospitalization was associated with colonization with ampicillin-resistant enterococci, while independent risk factors for nosocomial acquisition included treatment with more than three antibiotics, empirical use of antibiotics, use of third-generation cephalosporins and the use of enteral tube feeding. However, treatment with prophylactic antibiotics was not associated with vancomycin-resistant enterococci.

A crucial consideration for health-care professionals is the incidence of active tuberculosis in MICU patients. Frame and colleagues evaluated over 6000 admissions to the Henry Ford Hospital MICU between 1969 and 1984, where 61 (1%) of the patients had active tuberculosis with 43 (70%) of these presenting with acute respiratory failure. Predictive correlates included alcoholism in 51%, Gram-negative pneumonia, chronic obstructive pulmonary disease, prior tuberculosis, anti-tuberculosis medication non-compliance and malignancy[74]. The in-hospital mortality rate for all patients with tuberculosis requiring intensive care was 67%, but as high as 81% in those with acute respiratory failure.

Griffith and associates reported on the experience of 29 health-care workers exposed to an active case of unrecognized drug-susceptible pulmonary tuberculosis for 2 h in the emergency department and 10 h in the MICU[75]. Seventeen tuberculin skin-test-negative workers were followed, and 13 (76%) converted while 18% developed disease. This case illustrates the virulent nature of some organisms, mandating proper vigilance and precautions.

Pseudomonas cepacia was isolated as a cause of indolent bacteremia in 1988, associated with a 38% mortality rate, and was traced to a contaminated blood gas monitor[76].

High rates of septicemia (14–20%) were attributed to an epidemic incidence of *Serratia* and *Klebsiella* species in an analysis by Cortes and colleagues[77]. Disease patterns including epidemic presentation were identified in 6–14% of those admitted, with *Klebsiella* more regularly present than *Serratia* (27 day vs. 11 day LOS), but less virulent causing less septicemia (7% vs. 29%). Hence, the propensity to progress from indolent colonization to invasive iatrogenic infection is dependent on prevalence, virulence and host immune status.

Enterococcal bacteremia seems truly to afflict the most severely ill of the MICU patient population. Rimailho and colleagues reported on 35 patients with enterococcal bacteremia, noting a mean hospital stay of 17 ± 4 days, among whom 27 (77%) had experienced nosocomial acquisition, 20 (57%) received antibiotics, 16 (46%) had undiagnosed infectious focus, 13 (37%) had serious debilitating disease, and the deaths of nine (26%) were directly related to the bacteremia[78]. Better outcome was noted in those with nosocomial acquisition, those with appropriate antibiotic therapy early in the infection, and those without debilitation. The study recommendations are directed towards early diagnosis and empirical antibiotic therapy.

Gram-positive organisms are frequently noted to be ICU colonists. Crossley and Ross investigated colonizations in 92 medical and surgical ICU patients. *Staphylococcus aureus* was found in the pharynx, axilla, periurethral area and rectum equally frequently with and without nasal colonization, while *S. epidermidis* was found in all sites except the pharynx, and enterococci were commonly isolated from rectal sites[79]. The in-hospital strains appeared to be more virulent than those strains acquired in the community.

The nosocomial acquisition of *Candida albicans* can be a catastrophic outcome of in-patient care. Vazquez and co-workers prospectively defined the mechanism and risk factors associated with acquisition of *C. albicans* in 98 patients hospitalized on a bone marrow transplant unit, in whom surveillance cultures were performed[80]. *Candida albicans* was isolated from 52 (53%) of those studied, with 14 (14%) acquiring the organism after admission. A higher incidence of prior antibiotic use (92% vs. 64%) and length of time spent in the ICU (33 days vs. 13 days) were predictive of new *Candida* acquisition. Restriction enzyme analysis revealed 32 strain types, with four (12.5%) types common to 30 patients and 10 environmental surfaces. Identical strains of *C. albicans* were geographically and temporally associated, suggesting exogenous nosocomial acquisition through indirect patient contact.

Analysis of viral pathogens finds that respiratory syncytial virus (RSV) is a major cause of lower respiratory tract infection in children.

Guidry and co-workers evaluated a series of intubated adults in whom respiratory secretions were analyzed by all-culture and RSV enzyme immunoassay[81]. They found an extreme prevalence of disease: five of 11 (45%) intubated patients were culture positive; in addition, one of seven (14%) MICU employees and four of 48 (8%) ward patients had RSV-positive respiratory secretions. Thus, during community outbreaks of RSV infection, adult patients may be at risk for primary infection, and nosocomial infection is possible in other in-patients, transmitted by health-care personnel.

Various control and containment strategies have been suggested. Slaughter and colleagues evaluated the use of glove and gown precautions in 181 MICU patients, who presented with vancomycin-resistant enterococci in 14.8% of the control group and 16.1% of the treatment group[82]. There was no difference between levels of acquired vancomycin-resistant enterococci in the treatment (25.8%) and the control (23.9%) groups, with a mean time to colonization of 7.1–8.0 days. Risk factors for development of colonization included prolonged length of stay, enteral feeding and use of sucralfate.

An interesting perspective on barrier transmission precautions evaluates the likelihood of disease transmission from patient to health-care personnel. However, there may be a difference of clinical efficacy in protection from viral pathogens, depending on the product utilized. Kotilainen and associates reported a 2.5–10% incidence of penetration of herpes simplex virus type I across unused gloves using restriction endonuclease mapping[83]. However, the effectiveness of latex gloves, with a 1.4% (0–2.6%) failure rate in the 300-ml water tightness test, was significantly better than that of the vinyl version, with an 11.1% (4–28%) failure rate.

Investigation of further intervention modes will be required, as barrier methods have not proved effective in decreasing outbreaks of vancomycin-resistant enterococci.

Indwelling catheters

The increased use of triple-lumen catheters has been accompanied by an increase in sepsis. Ullman and co-workers performed daily culture of intraluminal fluid, demonstrating organisms in 14 of 31 (45%) catheters. This incidence was temporally related, and increased with increasing duration of catheterization beyond 7 days[84]. Hence, a weekly catheter change is appropriate for long-term indwelling catheters.

Bacteremia and sepsis

The incidence of bacteremia was 19% in a series of 574 MICU admissions, with 45% presenting in the first 48 h[85]. The clinical profile of those affected included older patients with longer ICU stays and a higher mortality rate (69% vs. 28%), compared to non-septic patients, especially for polymicrobial sepsis (91%) with shock. Patients were more commonly affected with Gram-negative than with Gram-positive (69% vs. 29%) organisms, associated with shock in 32%, and predisposition included decreased serum albumin for Gram-negative (but not Gram-positive) species, and the presence of intravascular catheterization with an airway as portal of entry. This profile may be helpful in predicting patients at risk.

Although recently discussed as a cost-saving measure, programs to limit the use of blood cultures have been described for a number of years. Gross and associates recommended a protocol that decreased the incidence of episodes of sepsis from 39 to 16% of patient discharges, and also decreased the mean number of blood cultures obtained from 1.2 to 0.3[86]. However, the practice pattern regressed to previous behavior when the protocol was stopped.

Scoring

Prognostic scoring systems have been adapted to give outcome prediction in septic shock patients. Baumgartner and colleagues reported the Simplified Septic Shock Score (SSSS), rating 13 clinical, biological and hemodynamic variables at admission, followed by the Complete Septic Shock Score (CSSS), additionally considering underlying disease states, characteristics of infection and microbiological data determined later in the disease course[87]. Their 88-patient derivation set documented a simplified score of 2.5 and 6.5 and a complete score of 3.1 and 8.4 in survivors and non-survivors, respectively (Tables 4 and 5). They found that both sepsis scoring systems performed better than the simplified acute physiology score (SAPS) or the APACHE II score.

Table 4 Simplified and complete septic shock scores. Table adapted from reference 87

Variable	*Points for calculating simplified septic shock score*				
	−2	−1	0	1	2
Clinical conditions					
Age (years)		< 65	65–69	≥ 70	
Sex (M/F)		M	F		
Mechanical ventilation		yes	no		
Glasgow coma scale (points)	< 13	—	≥ 13	—	—
Diuresis (ml/h)	—	< 20	≥ 20	—	—
Body temperature (°C)	< 37	—	37–39.5	≥ 39.5	
Histological values					
Hematocrit (%)	< 25	—	> 25	—	—
WBC count (cells/mm³)	—	< 1.5*	1.5–24.9*	25–39.9*	≥ 40
pH	< 7.10	7.10–7.24	7.25–7.49	—	≥ 7.50
Prothrombin time (s)	—	< 23	≥ 23	—	—
Hemodynamic values					
Heart rate (beats/min)	< 80	—	80–169	—	≥ 170
MAP (mmHg)	< 50	50–69	≥ 70	—	—
Cardiac index (l/min/m²)	<3.5	—	3.5–6.4	6.5–7.4	≤ 7.5

*Multiply by 10^3; WBC, white blood cell; MAP, mean arterial pressure

Therapy

Antibiotic usage for initial empirical treatment of infection in hospitalized patients was assessed by questionnaire in 82 medical or surgical ICUs by Knothe[88]. The most frequently used regimens for initial empirical therapy were first, combinations of broad-spectrum penicillin with an aminoglycoside, second, a second-generation cephalosporin with an aminoglycoside and third, a third-generation cephalosporin and an aminoglycoside.

Specific-use patterns included little empirical imipenem and fluoroquinolones, but more third-generation cephalosporins or imipenem–cilastin for MICU patients. In surgical ICU patients, the third-generation cephalosporins or broad-spectrum penicillin–amino-glycoside combinations were augmented by metronidazole in abdominal sepsis and peritonitis, and, for community-acquired

Table 5 Mortality rates for simplified and complete septic shock scores. Table adapted from reference 87

Points	Patients (*n*)	Deaths (*n*)	Mortality (%)
Simplified			
0	3	0	0
1	11	0	0
2	11	2	18
3	14	2	14
4	5	4	80
5	12	7	58
6	9	8	89
7	8	8	100
8	9	8	89
9	1	1	100
10	2	2	100
11	1	1	100
12	2	2	100
Complete			
0	2	0	0
1	8	0	0
2	10	1	10
3	12	1	8
4	4	1	25
5	9	3	33
6	6	3	50
7	12	12	100
8	7	6	86
9	3	3	100
10	6	6	100
11	3	3	100
12	4	4	100
13	1	1	100
14	1	1	100

pneumonia, by penicillin G, ampicillin or a second-generation cephalosporin with or without an aminoglycoside; the addition of clindamycin or metronidazole was described for staphylococcal infection or aspiration pneumonia.

GASTROINTESTINAL

The effectiveness of stress-ulcer prophylaxis is often debated in the critically ill. The etiology is often a combination of cellular dysoxia, excess acid production, ineffective neutralization and ischemia. In addition, there is a dearth of well-controlled studies defining therapeutic efficacy.

Ben-Menachem and co-workers evaluated 300 MICU patients, comparing the use of carafate and cimetidine to maintain gastric pH at < 4.0 with the outcome in control groups[89]. Stress-related gastritis was found to be equivalent in incidence in control (6%) and treatment (5%) groups. In addition, the patient groups had equivalent transfusion requirements, durations of MICU stay and mortality rates, suggesting the lack of efficacy of routine prophylaxis.

The risk of upper gastrointestinal bleeding after admission to the MICU was evaluated in 174 patients by Schuster and colleagues[90]. The overall rate of bleeding was 14%, and this group had higher mortality (64% vs. 9%), ICU length of stay (14 days vs. 4 days), mechanical ventilation requirement (84% vs. 26%) and duration of support (9 days vs. 4 days) than those who did not bleed. Factors associated with increased likelihood of bleeding included acute respiratory failure, malignancy and sepsis, while coagulopathy and the need for mechanical ventilation were most predictive. Therefore, prolonged mechanical ventilation (> 5 days), as opposed to a shorter duration (associated with a 3% bleeding rate), and coagulopathy are linked to the need for stress-ulcer prophylaxis.

Previously identified clinical criteria available at the time of triage have been evaluated in 103 MICU patients by Kollef and co-workers for their ability to predict outcome[91]. They classified 28 (27%) of the MICU admission to be at low risk for poor outcome. This group went on to have lower rates of recurrent gastrointestinal hemorrhage (3.6% vs. 27.5%), less acquired organ system dysfunction (1.0% vs. 1.5%), shorter lengths of hospital stay (4.9 days vs. 8.8 days), fewer units of blood transfused (1.3 vs. 6.2) and a lower overall mortality rate (0% vs. 21%), compared to high-risk admissions. Therefore, low-risk patients can be successfully triaged to less acute monitoring on an individual basis.

Another area of significant morbidity involves the onset of severe acute pancreatitis, occurring in 10–20% of cases. Deus and associates reported their experience of 319 such cases, of whom 51 (16%) had pancreatic effusions presenting as 14% effusion, 14% pseudocysts, 25% abscesses and 43% phlegmon[92]. The mortality rate was increased, compared to that of the general population (33% vs. 6%), and was worse still in those with alcoholic etiology, systemic complications and early surgical intervention, with a mortality rate of 40%.

HEPATIC

Generally, liver disease is particularly lethal in both acute and chronic conditions. Among deaths for which chronic liver disease was the underlying cause, 42% were associated with alcohol including cirrhosis and unspecified damage, 3% with chronic hepatitis, 1% with biliary cirrhosis and 53% with unspecified non-alcoholic conditions[93].

Turcotte and Child's classic description of postoperative mortality in cirrhotic patients with sepsis suggests that those with classification A (minimal severity) without biochemical or overt evidence of disease have a 0–10% mortality rate, those with class B (moderate severity) with bilirubin elevation and ascites have a 10–20% mortality rate and those with class C (severe) with hypoalbuminemia and encephalopathy have a 20–60% mortality rate. Thus, postnecrotic cirrhosis that results in portal hypertension is a significant adverse prognostic indicator (Table 6)[94].

Patients with hepatic failure admitted to the medical ICU generally have a poor prognosis. Shellman and colleagues retrospectively

Table 6 Postoperative mortality in those with sepsis. Table adapted from reference 94

| | Group designation | | |
Observation	A (minimal)	B (moderate)	C (advanced)
Serum bilirubin (mg/100 ml)	< 2.0	2.0–3.0	> 3.0
Serum albumin (g/100 ml)	> 3.5	3.0–3.5	< 3.0
Ascites	none	easily controlled	poorly controlled
Neurological disorder	none	minimal	advanced, 'coma'
Nutritional status	excellent	good	poor, 'wasting'
Postoperative mortality (%)	0–10	10–20	20–60

reviewed 100 MICU patients, demonstrating a 64% mortality rate, but univariate analysis found that 89% of Child's class C patients, 91% of those with assisted ventilation and 93% of those with creatine levels >1.3 mg/dl died during ICU stay, while multivariate analysis suggested 98% mortality if all three factors were present[95].

RENAL

The presence of renal failure and its influence on ICU outcome have been evaluated for patients that present with, or develop, renal dysfunction during their ICU stay.

Factors that may predispose patients to the development of renal failure were analyzed by Groeneveld and associates in a 487-patient sample, of whom 16% developed acute renal failure, with 63% treated with dialysis or renal replacement therapy and a 63% mortality rate[96]. Major independent factors contributing to increased mortality included advanced age, cardiovascular failure, pulmonary failure prior to acute renal failure and renal replacement therapy. The presence of chronic rather than acute renal failure was associated with fewer adverse effects, while sepsis had no influence.

However, the primary or secondary role of acute renal failure is unclear in that the same factors may cause both the renal failure and adverse outcome in survival, and they are co-variables and may not be causally linked.

Indicators identified to predict ICU outcome in those with renal failure have been derived by Schafer and co-workers, who examined 134 patients requiring dialysis in the MICU with an overall mortality rate of 57%[97]. Linear discriminate analysis correctly predicted outcome in 80% of patients beginning dialysis and in 85% at 48 h post-dialysis, identifying mechanical ventilation and hypotension as important predictive variables, comparing favorably with APACHE II outcome prediction in 58% of patients.

The predictability of acute renal failure can be enhanced by examining for the onset of sepsis, pancreatitis, bleeding, volume depletion, chronic liver disease, mechanical ventilation, central nervous system depression and surgery. The overall correct classification rate of the discriminate function was 78.5%, probably not enough to predict individual outcome[98].

Interestingly, the elderly with renal failure fare no worse than the general ICU population. Drum and colleagues evaluated 242 elderly (>65 years) patients with a 61% mortality rate: 49% in acute renal failure and 12% despite resolution of renal failure[99]. There was no difference when age was factored into the prediction model, with 57% mortality in those <18 years, 59% at 19–65 years, 60% at 65–68 years and 54% mortality in those >80 years. Outcomes were adversely affected by need for dialysis, creatine level >6 mg/dl, anuria, blood urea nitrogen level >120 mg/dl, ventilator dependence and septicemia. Although disease severity increased, mortality improved, decreasing from 70 to 50% as a result of aggressive care and monitoring developed between 1975 and 1990.

IMMUNOLOGY

It has been suspected that depressed cellular and humoral immunities are associated with a worsened outcome. Anergy, or lack of cell-mediated response to known antigens, can be associated with hemorrhage, massive transfusion and age over 60 years. Tasseau and co-workers evaluated 100 MICU patients with cutaneous antigen testing, demonstrating a 32% mortality rate for 49 anergic patients compared to 12% for the 51 reactive subjects[100].

Contact system activation has been examined as a prognostic marker in immune system response to infection or systemic inflammatory response syndrome. Pixley and colleagues observed 23 MICU patients while measuring contact activation system components including factor XII, prekallikrein, high-molecular-weight kinogen (HMW-K) factor XI, α2-macroglobulin kallikrein complex and factor V[101]. There was no admission difference documented, but survivors later demonstrated improvement in HMW-K and factor V levels during the recovery period.

Changes in plasma concentrations of vasoactive neuropeptides were measured by Arnalich and associates in 42 sepsis and control patients[102]. They found that calcitonin gene-related peptide and neuropeptide are released in sepsis, balancing the vasodilatation effects of the former and vasconstriction effects of the latter in compensated sepsis, while calcitonin gene-related peptide predominates in decompensated sepsis.

Pentoxifylline, a methylxanthine derivative, may alter serum cytokine concentrations and has been evaluated in therapeutic trials. Zeni and colleagues administered pentoxifylline in a 1 mg/kg bolus followed by infusion of 1.5 mg/kg/h for 24 h[103]. The serum tumor necrosis factor concentration was lower in the treatment groups than in the control group (12 pg/ml vs. 42 pg/ml), while the interleukin-6 and -8 levels were unchanged. Further study will be required to evaluate the clinical effect of decreasing this mediator in the setting of sepsis.

Mediators

Plasma levels of cytokines such as tumor necrosis factor-α (TNF-α), interleukin-1β (IL-1β), IL-6 and levels of endotoxins including lipo-polysaccharide (LPS) have been correlated with outcome by Casey and colleagues in 137 septic, critically ill and control patients[104]. They found that 54% of sepsis syndrome patients had detectable levels of TNF-α of 26 (0–1000) pg/ml, 37% had levels of IL-1 of 20 (0–2850) pg/ml, 80% had levels of IL-6 of 41.5 (0–2380) pg/ml and 89% had detectable levels of LPS of 2.6 (0–125) IU/l. These mediator levels were summarized as the total LPS–cytokine score, an increase in which was directly correlated with increasing mortality, independent of culture status. Although the IL-6 level was 69% higher in those who succumbed to sepsis, the wide range of response and the absence of a 'bright line' cut-off point between normal and abnormal levels limit the clinical utility of this technique at present.

Friedland and co-workers performed a similar analysis, measuring levels of pro-inflammatory cytokines TNF-α, IL-1β, IL-6 and IL-8 in 251 ICU patients. However, the drastic fluctuation in serious illness found no consistent relationship with bacteremia or systemic inflammatory response syndrome, and only admission IL-8 level or presence of TNF-α was an independent predictor of mortality[105].

The role of TNF-α in the pathogenesis of septic shock has been evaluated in 34 sepsis patients with a mortality rate of 61%, with one-quarter of these succumbing in the first 24 h[106]. The sepsis group had higher admission TNF-α levels (79 pg/ml vs. 0.5 pg/ml) as did the high-mortality group (917 pg/ml vs. 58 pg/ml), compared to the non-sepsis group and the lower-mortality group, respectively.

Lin and associates compared the relationship between plasma cytokine concentrations and leukocyte functional antigen expression in 40 patients[107]. Enzyme-linked immunosorbent assay revealed increased levels of IL-6, IL-8, IL-10 and TNF-α, and the cluster of differentiation (CD) 14+ monocytes measured by flow cytometry as a co-variable with IL-8 were lowest in those with severe sepsis. Thus, expression of specific functional molecules on peripheral blood leukocytes is variably related to the net production of certain monokines in sepsis.

HEMATOLOGY

Various hematological markers have been suggested to portend a poor prognosis in ICU patients, including anemia, neutropenia and thrombocytopenia.

The presence of thrombocytopenia as a marker for disseminated intravascular coagulation has been evaluated by Lee and co-workers in 107 MICU patients[108]. Thrombocytopenia was not found to be a risk factor in the general population. However, in the subgroup of patients with sepsis, 42% developed disseminated intravascular coagulation and 58% developed thrombocytopenia or a platelet count of < 150 000 × 10⁹/l, resulting in a 51% mortality. The platelet count in non-survivors of 97 × 10⁹/l was lower than that in survivors of 194 × 10⁹/l, and multiple regression analysis suggested that thrombocytopenia is an independent risk factor for mortality.

The presence of hematological malignancy is a significant adverse prognostic factor. Schuster and Marion's evaluation of 77 patients found an 80% overall hospital mortality rate, more often as a result of intractable hypotension than refractory hypoxemia[109]. Once respiratory failure develops in those with leukemia or lymphoma, remaining on mechanical ventilation as the result of infection for more than a brief period is associated with an adverse prognosis.

The issue of institution of life-support measures in this patient population was critically examined by Brunet and colleagues, who evaluated 260 patients and reported a 43% hospital and a 57% overall mortality[110]. This outcome was more favorable with 64% of patients still alive at 6 months and 44% by 1 year. However, the mortality rate in those who were hemodialyzed (67%) and mechanically ventilated (85%) was poor, and there were no long-term survivors if both conditions existed.

The short-term outcome of specific disease entities, such as leukemia and lymphoma, have been examined. Ashkenazi and co-workers retrospectively reviewed 29 patients: those with acute leukemia had a slightly better outcome, with seven of 21 (33%) surviving, than those with lymphoma, with two of 8 (25%) patients surviving[111]. The acute physiology score, rating 0–4 points for deviation from normal in several organ systems, was 28 ± 11, predicting a mortality of 56%; this was not significantly different from the actual mortality of 69%. Hence, the hematological malignancy and its effects on prognosis may not be separated from its associated physiological dysfunction.

A significant area of development is the effect of bone marrow transplantation on outcome. Paz and colleagues evaluated 43 admissions to the MICU for bone marrow transplantation, 77% of transplants being allogeneic (different genetic composition within the species) and 23% being autologous (similar genetic composition within the species)[112]. The ICU mortality rate was 67%, and similar for allogenic and autologous bone marrow transplantation. However, there was a clear discrepancy between a good-prognosis group, without the need for mechanical ventilation, with a shorter ICU stay (4.4 days) and a mortality rate of 3.7%, and a worsened-prognosis group, with the requirement of mechanical ventilation, a prolonged ICU stay (17.8 days) and a mortality rate of 81.3%. Thus, families should be counseled concerning outcome on the basis of mechanical ventilation requirement.

ONCOLOGY

The incidence of undiagnosed malignancy in patients presenting with the need for mechanical ventilation may be significant. Papadakis and colleagues retrospectively evaluated 172 autopsied patients cared for in the Veterans' Administration System, noting a 6% rate of extensive malignant neoplasm in non-survivors[113].

Sculier and Markiewicz evaluated 1413 patients admitted to the ICU of a specialty cancer unit in Brussels, of whom 1220 (86%) were admitted with solid tumors, mainly ovarian, breast and lung cancer, and 144 (10.2%) were admitted with hematological malignancies[114]. The overall mortality rate was only 10% but, with admission of acute medical emergencies in 621 (44%) cases for hypercalcemia accompanied by artificial ventilation, then 446 (72%) died during their ICU stay. A total of 732 (51.8%) were admitted to monitor special treatment or drug administration, including phase I drug infusion, intraperitoneal chemotherapy, use of a lipophilic drug containing liposomes and co-administration of platinum derivatives. Therefore, the oncological ICU not only provided acute care, but helped to optimize supportive care and development of new anticancer modalities.

The outcome of cardiopulmonary resuscitation has been examined in particular patient populations. Perhaps one of the worst prognostic categories is cardiac arrest in the oncology population. Sculier and Markiewicz performed a retrospective analysis of 49 cancer patients: initial cardiopulmonary resuscitation was successful in 19 (39%), but only five (10%) patients were discharged alive from the hospital[115]. Subgroup analysis found cardiopulmonary resuscitation to be successful in all eight cases of cardiovascular drug toxicity, even if the cancer was metastatic, while it was successful in only 25% of those patients with septic shock on respiratory failure. The conclusion was that in malignancy, as in most diseases, there is a better response to cardiopulmonary resuscitation with the more acute insult than with chronic decompensation.

RADIOLOGY

A significant proportion of early investigation concerning radiographic services concerned the use of the 'routine' daily chest X-ray. Strain and colleagues evaluated 507 consecutive radiographs in 94 MICU patients, 71 (14%) of which led to a management change[116]. Patients especially at risk, requiring unsuspected management changes, included those with cardiopulmonary instability and those requiring insertion of two or more catheters or tubes. Thus, previous recommendations suggest routine chest X-ray only for 'unstable' patients, and the problem of overuse can arise with lack of discrimination.

The efficacy of the daily portable chest X-ray was evaluated prospectively by Henschke and associates in 1132 consecutive radiographs in 140 patients[117]. The median number of chest radiographs was 0.7 per day; an artificial airway was present in 54% of patients with 12% malpositioned, and central venous catheters were present in 47% of patients with 9% malpositioned. There were significant interval changes in cardiopulmonary findings with use of portable radiography. For example, pneumothorax, lung collapse, infiltrate effusion or congestive heart failure was found in 44% of patients, although the actual clinical relevance of these findings was less certain.

However, the efficiency of the process comes into question. Greenbaum and Marschcall reported on a series of 200 radiographs, of which 74 (37%) were of suboptimal quality or performed after rounds too late for viewing, and, of the remainder, 54 (43%) revealed a new finding related to a device or disease process[118].

An additional consideration in the use of bedside radiography is the issue of radiation exposure. Boles and co-workers evaluated the dose to radiosensitive organs to define the 'average' patient, who was hospitalized for 9 days with six chest radiographs[119]. The average exposure was 292×10^{-5} Gy (mrad) to the sternal bone marrow, 239×10^{-5} Gy (mrad) to the thyroid gland, 3×10^{-5} Gy (mrad) to the testes and 1×10^{-5} Gy (mrad) to the ovaries for the chest and 605×10^{-5} Gy (mrad) to the eye for two maxillary sinus radiographs. Therefore, there was minor concern for patients involved in a long hospital stay, while dosimeters worn by the nurses measured to diffuse irradiation over a 2-month period.

Automated transmission and tracking systems for ICU radiographic images may vastly improve efficiency and physician effectiveness. Arenson and colleagues evaluated approximately 3000 portable chest X-ray examinations randomly assigned to digitalization compared to routine film archiving[120]. Approximately 65 radiographs were examined monthly and the time to major intervention, such as drug administration, decreased from 4.7 to 3.3 h with the use of this digital imaging technique; the immediate film availability had a beneficial effect.

A significant area of development in today's ICU is the radiological transition from film-based image to digital image management systems. Tucker and McEachern performed a quality assurance program evaluating 1082 examinations, and 87 (8.0%) of the digital images were associated with errors in practice, attributed to the interface between the information system and the operator[121].

In addition to diagnostic sensitivity, alterations to clinical practice effected by a change in radiological imaging system need to be considered. As mentioned above, Arenson and associates tracked 3000 portable chest X-rays performed in the MICU to find a decreased time to intervention in the digitalized system, compared to the conventional archiving system[120].

ENDOCRINE

The endocrine system, consisting of the hypothalamic–pituitary–endocrine axis, is often involved in multiple organ system dysfunction. The anterior pituitary axis includes the thyroid gland affected by thyroid stimulating hormone (TSH) to produce thyroxine (T_4); the ovary is stimulated by follicle stimulating hormone (FSH) and luteinizing hormone (LH) to produce estrogen and progesterone; the adrenal cortex is stimulated by adrenocorticotropic hormone (ACTH), melanocyte stimulating hormone and growth hormone to produce 17-ketosteroid, aldosterone and cortisol; and the breast is stimulated by prolactin. The posterior pituitary axis involves the release of vasopressin or antidiuretic hormone (ADH) affecting fluid homeostasis, and oxytocin targeting the uterus.

Critical illness commonly involves the adrenal, renal and thyroid systems in the ICU patient. Predisposing factors leading to adrenal insufficiency include spontaneous adrenal hemorrhage, often caused by heparin therapy, sepsis, hypotension, circulating anticoagulant or other stressful conditions[122].

Bouachour and associates evaluated 40 consecutive ICU patients by obtaining daily plasma cortisol levels and performing a short synthetic ACTH stimulation test within 24 h of admission[123]. The basal cortisol concentrations were increased, with 92% above 45 µg/dl and a mean of 36.8 µg/dl (range 7.9–113 µg/dl). There were no significant differences in outcome predicted by admission level of cortisol, although there was a slight increase noted at 72 h in non-survivors (66% vs. 38%). Similarly, there were no appreciable differences in the ACTH stimulation test between survivors and non-survivors to allow survival prediction.

Abnormalities in sodium and water balance are frequently present in those patients with severe illness. Lelarge and colleagues carried out an interventional study of 23 ICU patients with severe hyponatremia (Na < 120 mmol/l), which was associated with neurological dysfunction[124]. Patients had their water intake restricted, with sodium intake adjusted to natriuresis resulting in 'slow' correction of <12 mmol/l per 24 h in 16 cases and 'fast' correction of >12 mmol/l per 24 h in seven cases. After biochemical cure, two of seven patients undergoing fast correction had untoward outcome, including a death and central pontine myelinolysis. Therefore, caution is warranted in monitoring the speed of sodium correction.

Regulation of fluid balance also involves the osmolar receptor, where an increase in osmolarity causes activation of the ADH, sympathetic and renin–angiotensin–aldosterone systems to result in renal conservation of sodium and water to restore homeostasis.

Davenport and Zipser reported paradoxical suppression of plasma aldosterone, despite increased plasma renin activity in critically ill patients[125]. They found 22% of 100 ICU patients to have hyperreninemic and inappropriately reduced levels of plasma aldosterone, with the plasma aldosterone/renin ratio below the 98th centile. This group was affected by persistent hypotension (91% vs. 53%), compared to the normal group, resulting in related adrenal damage.

Thyroid disease is often discussed in the ICU setting as the 'sick-euthyroid' syndrome, with low levels of tri-iodothyronine (T_3) and T_4 and normal TSH. Melmed and colleagues compared 14 ICU patients with levels of T_4 <5.0 µg/dl with 99 patients with various medical conditions including pregnancy, cirrhosis and hypo- or hyperthyroid conditions[126]. Those with non-thyroidal illness were found to have decreased free T_4, elevated (reverse) RT_3 but normal or decreased TSH levels, while hyperthyroid patients were found to be differentiated by low RT_3 and high TSH levels.

The prevalence and clinical implications of hypocalcemia in acutely ill patients in a medical intensive care setting were studied in 88 patients by Desai and co-workers[127]. They found that 62 (70%) patients had decreased levels of both total and ionized calcium. The etiology of hypocalcemia was known in 28 (45%), including hypomagnesemia in 17 (28%), renal insufficiency in five (8%) alkalosis in four (6%) and acute pancreatitis in two (3%); however, there was no readily identifiable cause in 34 (55%) patients. Hypocalcemia was associated with a decrease in ionized calcium levels ($r = 0.33$) and total calcium levels ($r = 0.70$) and a septic state. The presence of hypocalcemia was associated with a significant increase in mortality (from 17 to 44%), compared to normocalcemic ICU patients. Thus, hypocalcemia is both commonly encountered and associated with a bad prognosis in the ICU setting.

VASCULAR

Perhaps one of the most significant issues in ICU care regarding disease surveillance and prophylaxis involves the proper diagnosis and therapy for deep venous thrombosis (DVT).

Hirsch and colleagues performed a surveillance study of 100 MICU patients using ultrasound with color Doppler imaging performed twice weekly, and 1 week after ICU discharge[128]. DVT was detected in 33% of patients with 48% lower- and 15% upper-extremity thrombosis. An unexpectedly high incidence occurred in patients despite prophylaxis in 61%, and yet the risk factors of age, gender, body mass index (BMI), cancer, surgery and duration of hospitalization failed to identify patients at risk.

Habscheid and associates performed a large-scale evaluation of DVT in 542 MICU patients who had routinely undergone ultrasound examinations[129]. Thromboses were demonstrated in 62 (11.4%) patients and were bilateral in 27.4%. DVT was most frequent (29%) in those with malignant disease and least frequent (3.7%) in those with myocardial infarction; autopsy revealed pulmonary embolism in 11 (13%) of the 87 patients evaluated. Therefore, careful diagnosis and early therapy is warranted in this population.

Interestingly, this high-prevalence population may not have commensurate prophylaxis. Keane and co-workers conducted a prospective survey of DVT prophylaxis in 152 MICU patients, and it was found that only 33% of those involved had adequate prophylaxis[130]. They remained in the ICU for 2.0 ± 2.8 days prior to institution of therapy where 87% had a single risk factor and 52% had multiple risk factors for DVT. Careful consideration is required as even this high-risk population is often undertreated.

RHEUMATOLOGY

The presence of rheumatological disease often contributes to severe systemic illness, resulting in significant adverse effects in hospitalized patients.

Godeau and colleagues evaluated 69 patients, 19 with rheumatoid arthritis (27.5%), 19 with necrotizing vasculitis (27.5%), 16 with systemic lupus erythematosus (23%), and 15 with other systemic rheumatic diseases (22%), with a mean age of 53 years and a SAPS of 12[131]. The principal reasons for admission were infection in 29 of 69 (42%), and acute exacerbation of rheumatological disease in 19 of 69 (27%). The mortality rate was 33% in the ICU and 42% by hospital discharge, mainly owing to infection with 83% acquired in the ICU. However, the mortality rate was no different for those patients with rheumatological disease than for a general ICU population with a similar SAPS score.

NUTRITION

The presence of malnutrition has an adverse effect on outcome in surgical patients, while less clear is the effect of nutritional repletion on improving survival.

Few investigators have examined outcome in medical patient populations. Muller and associates evaluated various total parenteral nutrition regimens, comparing hypocaloric (59 kJ/kg/day), isocaloric (117 kJ/kg/day) and hypercaloric (234 kJ/kg/day) nutrition and distribution of calories provided by varying carbohydrates, amino acids, and long- and medium-chain triglycerides administered within 2 days of the onset of multisystem organ failure in 20 critically ill (APACHE score 26) patients[132]. The mean energy expenditure was 130 kJ/kg/day, protein breakdown was 1.5 g/kg/day, temperature was 38°C, lactate level was 2.0 mmol/l and glucose level was 222 mg/dl. Carbohydrate administration did not prevent protein catabolism even with hypocaloric nutrition, nor did variations in triglyceride composition. The authors concluded that a hypocaloric (59 kJ/kg/day) diet with adequate protein (1.5 mg/kg/day) avoided the metabolic burden measured as increased energy expenditure, thermogenesis, urea production, glucose level and lactate level associated with iso- or hypercaloric diet.

The effectiveness of intensive nutritional regimens in patients who fail to wean from mechanical ventilation has been studied. Larca and Greenbaum compared 14 patients, eight of whom weaned successfully, and demonstrated that the groups did not differ in albumin level, transferrin level or lymphocyte count at study entry[133]. However, those that responded with successful weaning demonstrated an increase in both albumin and transferrin levels, compared to those who failed to wean.

NEUROLOGY

There is a wide range of neurological disturbance that can result in requirement of critical care monitoring and intervention. Primary disease such as delirium or coma, cerebrovascular event, myopathy and neuropathy, and infectious conditions such as meningitis or encephalitis can result in ICU admission. Likewise, these disease entities can also occur as a secondary process arising during the ICU course itself.

Coma

The outcome of patients who suffer cardiac arrest and post-anoxic encephalopathy is of crucial importance. Abramson and colleagues reported the prehospital arrest experience of 262 comatose victims, evaluating arrest time and duration of cardiopulmonary resuscitation (Table 7)[134]. If the arrest time was brief (<6 min) and the duration of cardiopulmonary resuscitation was prolonged (>30 min), the chance of good outcome was only 3%. However, if the arrest time was prolonged (>6 min) and the duration of cardiopulmonary resuscitation was prolonged (>15 min), the chance of good outcome was 0%.

The outcome of hypoxic–ischemic coma in 210 hospitalized patients was reported by Levy and co-workers, and 13% of patients regained independent function at some point during the first post-arrest year[135]. Absence of pupillary light reflex on examination precluded return to ordinary function. Those with pupillary light reflex, development of spontaneous eye movement and withdrawal from pain regained independence in 41% of cases (Table 8).

Diagnostic modalities used to assist in prognostication in patients with anoxic encephalopathy have been explored in a variety of contexts. Invasive modalities include the monitoring of jugular bulb oxygenation,

Table 7 Post-anoxic encephalopathy outcome: prehospital arrest experience. Table adapted from reference 134

Arrest time (min)	*CPR duration* (min)	*Good outcome* (%)
< 6	< 30	50
< 6	> 30	3
> 6	< 5	50
> 6	> 15	6

CPR, cardiopulmonary resuscitation

Table 8 Post-anoxic encephalopathy outcome: in-hospital experience. Table adapted from reference 135

Function	Patients (n)	Performance	Good outcome (%)
Initial	210		
Pupillary light reflex		absent	0
1 day	168		
Motor withdrawal		absent	1
Spontaneous eye movement		absent	
3 days	124		
Motor withdrawal		absent	0
1 week	76		
Obey command		absent	0
Spontaneous eye movement		absent	0
2 weeks	61		
Oculocephalic reflex		absent	0
One of			
obey command		no	
spontaneous eye opening		no	
eye opening improvement 2 grades		no	

currently being explored for benchmark data. Van der Hoeven and associates evaluated 13 patients who were comatose after prehospital cardiac arrest, but oxygen saturation, extraction ratio and lactate difference could not discriminate those with good from those with adverse prognostic outcome[136]. This area is certainly exciting and will require further investigation in larger patient groups.

Non-invasive prognostication strategies have traditionally advised on electroencephalographic assessment of anoxic injury. Madl and colleagues recently evaluated the predictive ability of sensory evoked potential to predict outcome in 441 adult, non-traumatic comatose patients, defined as unarousable, unresponsive to stimuli or Glasgow coma scale score of < 7[137]. The worse-prognosis group (20%) had bilateral loss of cortical evoked potential peak N20, and 100% succumbed without awakening. The better-prognosis group, with preserved cortical N20 peak, exhibited 42% survival. It was found that a preserved N20 peak was not useful in predicting individual survival, with an N13–N20 conduction time of >7 ms demonstrating a positive predictive value of 0.67, while the absence of this peak could reliably predict adverse outcome (Table 9).

Polyneuropathy

The onset of significant sensorimotor weakness in the critically ill ICU patient has been described as the critical illness polyneuropathy.

Hund and colleagues performed electrodiagnostic studies in seven ICU patients from 3 weeks to 3 years, demonstrating a clinical pattern of moderate to severe limb weakness with marked atrophy, and with some decrease in, but preservation of, deep tendon reflexes[138]. Electromyography demonstrated severe acute denervation of proximal muscles; muscle and nerve biopsies revealed severe neurogenic atrophy and axonal degeneration without inflammation. The mortality rate was two of seven (29%) patients, but those that recovered did so completely although retaining signs of chronic neurogenic damage.

Therefore, the critical illness polyneuropathy is a syndrome affecting proximal, facial and paraspinal musculature, with reflexes that are slightly decreased with lower motor neuron disease and exaggerated with upper motor neuron lesions. Clinical recovery is usually rapid

Table 9 Diagnostic analysis

Sensitivity	$\dfrac{TP}{TP + FN}$
Specificity	$\dfrac{TN}{TN + FP}$
Accuracy	$\dfrac{TP + TN}{TP + TN + FP + FN}$
Positive predictive value	$\dfrac{TP}{TP + FP}$
Negative predictive value	$\dfrac{TN}{TN + FN}$

TP, true positives; FN, false negatives; TN, true negatives; FP, false positives and complete after the ICU course, while electrophysiological testing and histological evidence may lag behind clinical recovery, especially in the peroneal nerve.

TOXICOLOGY

A notable proportion of medical intensive care is directed towards the management of toxicological emergencies.

The most common overdose occurring in a series of 53 patients admitted to the MICU involved tricyclic antidepressant agents in 50% of cases, followed by barbiturates in 20%[139]. Interestingly, 25% of intentional overdoses were free of psychiatric disease, while unintentional overdoses occurred more commonly in substances abusers.

Another problematic overdose is propoxyphene. Sloth-Madsen and co-workers described the experience of 222 patients, with 73% presenting with neurological symptoms: 10% convulsions, 48% impaired circulation or shock, and 45% respiratory failure[140]. A mortality rate of 8% was observed. Twelve patients (5%) presented in asystole, half of whom were resuscitated without sequelae. The authors recommended a 24-h arrhythmia-free interval before ICU discharge.

Early experience with acute poisoning was reported by Kallenbach and associates, who described 103 patients admitted to the MICU, comparing only 6.1% of poisoning cases overall with an associated 5.8% mortality rate[141].

Heyman and colleagues reported on 43 intentional drug-overdose patients, with the majority surviving (95%) after presenting with a GCS of 12.5 (range 3–15) and an APACHE II score of 8 (range 1–29)[142]. Clinical presentation included mechanical ventilation requirement in 12%, while 4% had serious electrocardiographic changes. The vast majority of overdose patients, therefore, do not require ICU care, which should be reserved for those with significant neurological dysfunction or cardiac abnormality.

The use of gastric lavage in emergency department patients has been associated with a higher prevalence of MICU admission, usually owing to aspiration pneumonia.

Stern and colleagues performed a comprehensive evaluation of 255 patients responsible for 283 admissions, 5% of the total for drug overdose[143]. Post-hospitalization study found that 8% died subsequently,

5% by overdose, while 42% had been readmitted for another non-fatal overdose or psychiatric illness. Prior psychiatric treatment was associated with subsequent readmission; 61% of those with a history of suicide attempts were readmitted to the MICU. This predictive model may be helpful, considering the high personnel and societal costs associated with repeat overdose admissions.

Deliberate repeat self-poisoning is a common problem in the drug-overdose population. Ojehagen and associates interviewed 59 patients, 1 year after a MICU stay for deliberate overdose, from an original group of 79 admissions[144]. Successful suicide attempts were completed by two (3.4%) patients, while 16 (27%) demonstrated repeat suicidal behavior. These repeaters more commonly had incurred alcohol abuse, dysthymia (diagnostic and statistical manual of mental disorders grade III (DSM-III), axis I) diagnosis, previous suicide attempts and ongoing treatment. In fact, half of the patients remained in treatment, while yet repeating earlier failed self-poisoning attempts.

The social costs of substance abuse-related admissions to adult MICUs and surgical ICUs are significant. Baldwin and co-workers reported on 435 ICU admissions, of which 14% were tobacco-related generating 16% of costs, 9% were alcohol-related responsible for 13% of costs and 5% were illicit drug-related generating 10% of costs[145]. The net effect was that substance abuse-related events accounted for 28% of all ICU admissions, were responsible for 39% of costs and resulted in longer (4.2 days vs. 2.8 days) and more expensive ($US 9610 vs. $US 5890) hospital stays, compared to other general ICU admissions. The uninsured group was found to have 44% of its admissions related to substance abuse and generating 61% of all costs.

There is no simple solution to this difficulty, but public empowerment and education may provide a partial answer.

PHARMACOLOGY

The development of pharmacology services has progressed beyond simple analysis of drug pharmacokinetics and pharmacodynamics to assisting in all aspects of effectiveness and efficiency of drug administration.

The patterns of medication use in the MICU were evaluated by Smythe and colleagues in 1993[146]. The mean length of stay for ICU patients was 5.2 ± 9.8 days, the mean age was 62.7 years and the overall mortality rate was 33%. Survival was adversely affected in those older (69 years vs. 63 years), post-cardiopulmonary resuscitation, suffering a stroke, or with APACHE II > 19. The mean daily number of medications was 7.5 ± 3.4 and the total number was 12.1 ± 7.6 drugs. The most commonly administered types of medication were anti-hypertensives or vasodilators in 69% and gastrointestinal prophylaxis agents in 65%. There was a positive linear relationship between length of stay and number of medications used, as well as those used in non-survivors.

Careful management of the multiplicity of pharmacological agents utilized in the ICU setting may improve medication effectiveness while monitoring costs. Traditionally, there have been attempts to monitor clinical effectiveness of pharmacology input by examining drugs with predictable pharmacokinetic profiles, such as aminoglycosides and antiepileptic drugs.

Dager and Albertson evaluated the effectiveness of a clinical pharmacist in monitoring theophylline levels in a control group (11 patients) and a treatment group (14 patients), for which the pharmacist plotted pharmacokinetic data to plan therapy[147]. There were 27 theophylline rate changes and 1.01 ± 0.3 levels ordered in the physician control protocol, while there were 44 rate changes with 0.62 ± 0.3 levels ordered in the treatment protocol. The authors found that both inappropriate medication concentration and number of emergency requests decreased with this protocol.

The effect of interventions by a pharmacist and nurse on the cost of drug therapy in a MICU has been evaluated by Katona and colleagues. In this study, the pharmacist taught cost-avoidance techniques to the nursing staff[148]. Most of the interventions resulted in discontinuation of medications or changes in drug use of antimicrobial agents, saving $US 6383 in direct cost avoidance and $US 23 993 in projected cost avoidance for the duration of therapy.

PSYCHIATRY

Psychiatric dysfunction can occasionally result in ICU stay secondary to drug overdose, abuse or withdrawal, associated with endocrine dysfunction or presentation of acute delirium.

A potentially catastrophic outcome of the use of psychotropic agents is the neuroleptic malignant syndrome presenting with hyperpyrexia, altered consciousness, muscular rigidity and movement dysfunction[149]. This is a rare idiosyncratic reaction secondary to therapeutic and non-toxic medication dosing, usually of phenothiazines, but also of butyrophenones and thioxanthenes (haloperidol or fluphenazine). The disease is often associated with leukocytosis, elevated creatine phosphokinase and liver enzyme elevations, with a mortality rate of approximately 20%, and should be included in the differential diagnosis of the febrile patient with rigidity and prior neuroleptic use.

Another consideration is the unrecognized drug dependence in psychiatrically hospitalized elderly patients. Whitcup and Miller analyzed a series of 90 patients to define 19 (21%) as being drug dependent. Half of these patients had been unrecognized as such, and the majority (seven of ten) experienced serious medical complications[150]. The demographic profile suggested that most women were dependent on benzodiazepines, while men were more likely to be alcohol abusers.

Confusion in patients is frequently undetected by nurses, owing to superficial patient interviews. Scherubel and Tess evaluated the Mini-Mental State Examination, Clinical Assessment of Confusion, and a Visual Analog Scale of Confusion, which were administered to 53 critically ill patients[151]. All three grading scales correlated with clinical assessment on more than 75% of the study days.

The psychosocial aspects of ICU recovery are a critical component of outcome. Schilling and colleagues interviewed 54 patients using two rating scales and psychopathological findings (AMDP system)[152]. There were wide variations with few systemic trends, indicating individualized coping strategies. However, the reaction to ICU admission remembered later on the general ward was almost uniform: threat to life was minimized and personal capabilities enhanced. Systematically colored recollections are seen as a part of further coping strategies, restoring the individual competence of coping and minimizing the offense of illness.

Sleep deprivation is often a precipitating factor in decompensation of cognitive function in the ICU patient. Edwards and Schuring attempted to validate staff nurses' observations of sleeping and waking states using polysomnography in 21 adult patients[153]. There were 17, 15-min observation periods per patient, and the nurses' assessment of sleep state was correct 82% of the time. Therefore, nursing observations are a very reliable means of determining whether the patient is at risk for sleep deprivation.

The needs of family members of ICU patients are often underappreciated, as they react differently to the stress of hospitalization of a loved one. Cray described the use of a clinical nurse specialist to provide structured, individualized support to families of the critically ill[154]. This intervention received positive reactions from both the family and the primary nurse involved in the care plan.

Comprehensive ICU management requires that the psychological needs not only of the patients but also of the families are addressed. Perez-San Gregorio and co-workers evaluated 76 gravely traumatized patients and their families, and found that more than 50% of family members of trauma ICU patients showed symptoms of depression; women especially demonstrated hypochondria, suicidal ideation, anxiety, low energy, guilt, resentment, apathy–withdrawal, paranoia, schizophrenia and psychasthenia[155]. They concluded that the psychological characteristics of the trauma families were far from the normal adjustment of the control group.

Henneman and associates devised a trial of information communication to ICU patient family members[156]. They questioned family members 24–48 h into their loved one's ICU course about their knowledge of unit policies and personnel, manipulating two variables:- flexible visiting hours and information booklets. Obviously, those families who were the most satisfied and informed were those who had been allocated the educational program.

SURGERY

Occasionally, patients admitted to the ICU with medical conditions will go on to require surgical intervention. Lerch and colleagues evaluated 1024 patients referred to a general MICU, of whom 7% went on to have emergency surgery[157]. They used ultrasound as a diagnostic adjunct in 25% of cases, especially in hemorrhage (44%), septicemia (39%) or disease of the urinary tract (56%).

Kollef and Allen evaluated 1617 medical ICU patients to identify 4% who developed an acute abdominal process amenable to surgical intervention[158]. The mortality rate of 16% of these patients that did not undergo surgery was 100%, compared to 25% mortality in those who underwent surgical intervention. They used two factors, an organ system failure index of >2 and an APACHE II score of >18, to identify subsets at risk, with 5% surgical mortality if neither factor was present and 84% if both were present.

The outcome of surgical intervention for intra-abdominal catastrophe in the MICU patient is predictable based on rapidity of diagnosis, intervention and associated organ system involvement or physiological disturbance.

MATERNAL–FETAL MEDICINE

An infrequent but potentially catastrophic occurrence is the presence of critical illness during pregnancy. Kirshon and co-workers evaluated maternal mortality over a 6-year period, with a maternal mortality rate of 21.7/100 000 or ten maternal deaths in 45 984 deliveries[159]. However, after development of an obstetric ICU staffed by maternal–fetal medicine specialists, and obstetric anesthesiologists established in the labor and delivery suites, the rate progressed to 22.1/100 000 or 11 maternal deaths in 49 700 deliveries. This mortality appeared to be predominately caused by hypertension, hemorrhage and infection. The authors found this care to be equivalent to that traditionally provided by medical intensive care specialists.

Owing to a paucity of literature concerning ICU care of the obstetric patient, Collop and Sahn reviewed the findings of 20 obstetric patients admitted to the MICU, compared to non-obstetric controls[160]. The obstetric population contained 10 (50%) patients with pre-existing medical problems, and had a maternal mortality rate of 20% and a fetal mortality rate of 35%. All maternal deaths were accompanied by ARDS and respiratory failure, but were also accompanied by equivalent rates of mechanical ventilation. This group is clearly at high risk with accompanying maternal and fetal mortality.

CONTINUOUS QUALITY IMPROVEMENT

An effective MICU design requires an effective quality assurance or continuous quality improvement program to ensure medical standards, development of new therapeutic plans and improvement in health care delivered.

Quality assessment and assurance require systemic monitoring and evaluation of patient care, oriented to reflect changes dependent on patient type, age and length of stay. Sivak and Perez-Trepichio's model for analysis developed at Cleveland Clinical Hospital grouped data into structural, process and outcome categories[161]. They further stressed in a follow-up study the need to establish indicators of quality, gather data and then organize data into useful information[162]. Their model focused on the structure process and outcome of patient care, applying the concept of patient days of service to quantify utilization of resources.

Before quality of care can be assessed, the end-points must be defined. Each practitioner's performance should be evaluated for technical and interpersonal aspects[163]. The standard of technical performance is judged in comparison with the 'best in practice', defined as being associated with the greatest improvement in health. The 'effectiveness' or realized fraction of what is achievable is based on the summation of technical performance to attain the desired therapeutic end-point. Interpersonal exchange provides information about the nature of illness and its management, motivating the patient's collaboration in their care, noted as 'measures of quality-adjusted life'.

OUTCOME

Prediction models

The most widely used outcome prediction models include the acute physiology and chronic health evaluation (APACHE), simplified acute physiology score (SAPS) and mortality prediction model (MPM). They are helpful and allow some general sense of performance by disease category, but are less successful at predicting individual patient outcome, as well as requiring computer assisted methodology.

The APACHE system is the most widely utilized grading system in the medical ICU setting. Kruse and colleagues compared the predictive accuracy of the APACHE system with clinical assessment by critical-care personnel on admission of 366 patients[164]. They found that mortality prediction was similar for all groups: fellows, residents, interns, nurses and the APACHE II system. However, the area under the receiver operating characteristic (ROC) curve was improved for the fellows, compared to the nurses (0.89 vs. 0.84).

The accepted scoring systems have been compared for accuracy. Schafer and associates analyzed both a general ICU population and a group from which cardiac patients were excluded, compared the MPM, APACHE II and SAPS systems[165]. The sensitivity or correct prediction of hospital mortality was 45%, 51% and 21%, respectively; specificity or correct prediction of hospital survival was 84%, 85% and 97%, respectively; overall accuracy or correct classification rate was 74%, 76% and 76%, respectively. Slightly improved sensitivity was found in the non-cardiac ICU population, but decreased accuracy measured as goodness of fit was found, compared to those with cardiac disease.

There were marked inconsistencies between estimated risk and observed mortality, limiting applicability for grading of individual illness and outcome. The major utility is for global comparisons of ICU populations. Meaningful comparison of patient outcomes requires a measure of severity of illness to improve predictive ability. Gross and co-workers compared the APACHE II system, the accepted benchmark indicator for disease severity, with the computerized severity score and three simpler predictors, the co-morbidity, McCabe–Jackson and American Society of Anesthesiologists scoring systems[166]. They found that all scoring systems correlated well as comparable predictors of co-morbidity in the MICU, and suggested that some modification would improve the performance of the standard scoring system.

The APACHE II score has been examined as a marker for physiological stress in the acutely ill. Brown and colleagues used indirect calorimetry to define a relationship between increasing APACHE II score measured and true resting energy expenditure[167]. However, the relationship was sufficiently weak ($r^2 = 0.12$–0.23) to suggest that the APACHE II score should not be substituted for indirect calorimetry assessment of stress state in certain patients who are critically ill.

Multisystem organ failure is the most common cause of death in critically ill medical patients. Tran and associates evaluated 487 MICU patients retrospectively, reporting a 28% incidence of single system organ failure with a mortality rate of 16%, and a 38% incidence of multisystem organ failure associated with a 58% mortality rate[168]. The overall mortality rate of 27% was determined by advanced age, chronic disease and number of failing organs, particularly the cardiovascular, pulmonary, renal and neurological systems.

There have been attempts to provide ICU specific outcome predictors. Kollef utilized logistic regression analysis in 277 MICU, surgical ICU and cardiothoracic ICU patients to identify independent predictors of mortality, removing the organ system failure index >3 as a confounding variable[169]. Factors associated with mortality in the MICU included renal failure; in the surgical ICU supine head positioning, acute physiology score >10, and preadmission life-style score >2; and in the cardiothoracic ICU requirement of acute dialysis, ventilator-associated pneumonia and occurrence of an iatrogenic event.

The site of hospital admission was considered to be an independent prognostic factor. Escarce and Kelley evaluated 235 patients, reporting a mortality rate of 22% in those admitted from the emergency department, 36% for those transferred from other hospitals, 55% in those coming from the hospital floor and 59% in those from the medical intermediate care unit[170]. Logistic regression analysis confirmed an independent association between mortality rate and site of admission independent of APACHE II score, which underestimated mortality in all but the emergency department groups.

Clinical

General prediction strategies have been suggested by individual patient samples, such as worsened outcome with sepsis, age or stroke, compared to the general population, based on an analysis by Lee and colleagues, indicating a 37% MICU mortality rate[171]. Practitioners attempt to predict individual patient outcome based on a disease-specific historical classification generally with moderate success.

Brannen and co-workers compared physician assessment with APACHE II score in outcome prediction, and found that the human clinical prediction performed significantly better than the computer model[172]. They suggested a Bayesian theorem-based system, modifying prediction based on prevalence, resulting in better performance with a predicted mortality risk of <30%.

Christensen and associates compared MICU survival estimates of physicians and nurses with those based on the APACHE II system[173]. The MICU personnel were fairly accurate discriminators of survival; although consistent underestimation occurred, accuracy improved with level of training during the initial 24 h. Physicians seemed to be better at prediction, while the APACHE II system performed better in terms of discrimination.

NURSING

The presence of a collaborative-care model involving both nurses and physicians working in a co-operative strategy is an important part of effective ICU care. Youngner and colleagues, in an early evaluation of the ICU work environment, found in a poll of 36 house officers and 34 nurses that the nurses were less satisfied with the decision-making and communication processes of the critical care area[174]. They suggested four methods to optimize care in the medical ICU by:

(1) Recognizing the inevitability of conflict in a system where physicians have ultimate authority;

(2) Avoiding the perpetuation of stereotypes;

(3) Maximizing the continuity of physician care;

(4) Optimizing communication between professional groups.

The Rush unification model aids in the development of clinical practice by nursing education, suggesting a teaching and clinical appointment-encouraging collaboration to achieve goals[175].

The protocolized care plan or 'care map' has been utilized to care for those with diabetic ketoacidosis in the intensive care setting by an interdisciplinary team, with good results[176].

This interdisciplinary collaboration has been examined by Baggs and colleagues in an assessment of the subjective reports of house staff and nurses[177]. Nurses' reports of collaboration were positively associated with patient outcome: predicted risk of negative outcome decreased from 16% when nurses reported on collaboration in decision-making to 5% when the process was fully collaborative. However, this finding did not extend to physician reporting of collaboration and partial outcome.

Another important consideration is the effect of nursing intervention on hospital efficiency and effectiveness. The therapeutic intervention scoring system (TISS) quantifies the amount and extent of health-care resources required, based on ICU intervention[178]. The TISS score has been validated as predictive of outcome, as well as of ICU resources necessary for patient care. Adam and colleagues examined a medical ICU population with a 23% mortality rate overall, among whom non-survivors had a higher admission TISS score (mean 20) while survivors had a lower discharge score (mean 5)[179]. Staffing considerations based on 24 TISS points a day per nurse were more reliable than bed-occupancy considerations based on a two-patient-per-nurse staffing model.

However, the most useful analysis would examine the effect of nursing care on outcome based on length of stay or mortality. Thorens and co-workers evaluated the effect of nursing on 15 patients with chronic obstructive pulmonary disease requiring mechanical ventilation and 72 historical controls, measured as the 'index of nursing', comparing the effective and ideal work-force based on nursing number and qualifications[180]. A significant inverse correlation existed between duration of mechanical ventilation and nursing index. As the nursing index increased to 1.05, where 1.0 indicated adequate staffing, the duration of ventilation decreased from 38.2 ± 25.8 to 9.9 ± 13 days. Thus, the duration of weaning would increase significantly in an understaffed ICU.

BED UTILIZATION

A survey of ICU bed use was offered by Singapore General Hospital for 112 patients admitted with pulmonary disease (63%)[181]. The mean duration of stay was 7.2 ± 1.5 days for sepsis and 4.7 ± 0.5 days for other diagnoses, and there was increased mortality in the septic group (43% vs. 37%).

The common presumption is that admissions are related to the number of available beds. However, Kelley and associates prospectively analyzed MICU admissions after a 100% increase in bed availability but found no resultant change in ICU occupancy, length of stay, hospital and ICU mortality or readmission rate[182]. Thus, extra bed availability did not translate into inappropriate increased bed utilization.

A significant proportion of resources is devoted to generating admission or discharge criteria for the ICU, encouraging more efficient bed utilization. However, the subject of ICU admission criteria has not been carefully studied. The American College of Physicians' Clinical Efficacy Assessment Project analyzed 970 articles pertinent to critical care, with only two case–control studies that directly measured the effect of ICU intervention on mortality[183]. This lack of concrete admission and outcome data will require decision-making models to be validated by prospective randomized trials.

Most of the analysis in this area has examined discharge criteria. Attempts have been made to identify clinical variables associated with unexpected death or readmission to the MICU. Rubins and Moskowitz evaluated 300 consecutive patients, comparing those with and without complications during their hospital stay[184]. They found from multivariate analysis that age, acute physiology score on admission and diagnosis of upper gastrointestinal bleeding were independent predictors of unexpected adverse outcome and unit readmission. Presence of these risk factors may warrant closer and more prolonged observation.

The use of consensus guidelines may help to minimize individual practice variations. Eagle and colleagues evaluated 1145 consecutive MICU admissions for the effect of physician feedback on length of stay, with a decrease in hospital stay from 7.4 to 7.1 days, and ICU stay from 2.5 to 2.1 days[185].

Studies attempting to improve ICU bed utilization stress early-discharge strategies. Bone and co-workers analyzed 1492 articles pertinent to ICU discharge, identifying only two studies that distinguished low-risk populations[186]. Clearly, a definitive low-risk category of potential ICU patients could improve overall effectiveness.

Consideration of alternatives to standard intensive or coronary care beds is necessary to utilize available resources optimally. The use of non-intensive care telemetry has been suggested to conserve critical care resources. Estrada and colleagues evaluated 2240 patients admitted to a telemetry unit for chest pain (55%), arrhythmia (14%), heart failure (12%) and syncope (10%); direct modification of management occurred in 7% and was reviewed as useful, but no action was taken based on new information on management in 5.7%[187]. Clinical deterioration occurred in 39% of patients with a 0.9% mortality rate of admissions; four of the 20 deaths occurred during monitoring, while 11 were transferred to the ICU. Effective utilization of telemetry requires vigilance to predict early deterioration, to prevent a catastrophic event.

Another resource that has been explored is the non-invasive respirator care unit (NRCU), a distinct unit generally used to deliver intensive respiratory therapy, avoiding mechanical ventilation. Elpern and associates evaluated 136 patients admitted to a respiratory care unit where costs exceeded charges by $US 1.5 million annually, with losses greatest for those requiring mechanical ventilation, or those with Medicare and Medicaid as primary payers[188]. However, the daily costs were decreased (by $US 1976) in the NRCU, compared to the MICU. Thus, the NRCU can help to minimize losses for the critically ill requiring aggressive pulmonary toilet to avert endotracheal intubation. Perhaps the area attracting the most attention is the use of the intermediate or progressive care unit to provide titrated nursing and physician care.

A model to predict the probability of requiring life-supporting therapy has been explored in 8040 patients by Zimmerman and colleagues[189]. The most important determinants of requirement for life-supporting therapy were the diagnosis, acute physiology component of the APACHE III score, age, operative status, patient location and hospital length of stay before ICU admission, suggesting that 77% had a low (<10%) risk of receiving active treatment during the ICU stay. Therefore, an isolated low-risk group may benefit from an intermediate care stay, avoiding the potential iatrogenic hazards of an ICU stay.

Interestingly, individual institutions have gone full cycle with the presence, absence and return of the progressive care unit. Byrick and co-workers examined the effects of intermediate care area closure on the admission strategies of 217 patients[190]. They found an increase in non-emergent coronary care unit admission (from 4 to 11%) and a decrease in APACHE II score (from 22 to 19), resulting in an increase in proportion (from 5 to 13%) of those with minor (APACHE score < 15) illness in the critical care unit.

The success of the individual unit is based on versatility and the ability to titrate rapidly the staff who are delivering care.

ETHICS

The issues of patient autonomy, family-substitute decision-making and futility of care are paramount considerations in end-of-life decision-making.

Both patients and families ($n = 160$) who had experienced medical intensive care were willing to undergo additional ICU care, in 70% of cases to achieve 1 additional month of survival, while 8% were unwilling to undergo care for any prolongation of survival[191]. Personal preferences were clearly in conflict with public policy matters, as preferences were poorly correlated with functional status, quality of life, life expectancy, age, severity of critical illness, length of stay or charges.

The frequency of advanced directives is poor, with only 8.8–11.3% presenting with written documentation even after implementation of the Patient Self-Determination Act (PSDA) from Johnson and associates' series of 204 patients[192]. Although a significant amount of discussion takes place regarding advanced directives, they are often unavailable or not followed by family members.

Early discussions of support limitation were held only infrequently with prospective family members. Blackhall and colleagues reported the experience of 611 patients admitted to the MICU of a tertiary-care teaching hospital and found that a 'do not resuscitate' status was discussed in only 11% of cases and more frequently in those who were older, more critically ill, of poor intellectual function and admitted to the MICU as opposed to the critical care unit[193].

Youngner and co-workers published a survey of 'do not resuscitate' decisions in a series of 506 patients, of whom 71 (14%) were designated DNR and 69 (13%) went on to survive[194]. This group could be predicted by severity of illness, age and prior health, and consumed a significant proportion of resources. The justification for 'do not resuscitate' decision-making included poor prognosis (59%), poor quality of life (24%) and patients' wishes (15%), with no written justification for 42%.

Another common misconception is that invocation of end-of-life maneuvres is usually used in cases of treatment futility. Halevy and colleagues evaluated 129 patients and found relatively few resources consumed by unrecoverable patients[195]. There were only 2 bed-days (0.3%) used for those with 90% predicted mortality, 22 bed-days (3.6%) used for those with hypoxic ischemia coma and 10 bed-days (1.6%) used for those with the five established lethal conditions. Grouping these 'futile' treatment conditions resulted in a total resource consumption rate of 20.3%, an appreciable but not overwhelming proportion of cases.

Methodology to deal with ethical decision-making in the nursing-home population is desirable. Kellogg and Ramos reported on their experience with 350 nursing-home residents: status was decided in 80% of patients, and mostly by surrogates (73%) 'do not resuscitate' orders (80%)[196]. After a 'do not resuscitate' decision, neither the care intensity nor the hospital use changed in this group marked by dementia, white race and older age. Those with 'do not resuscitate' orders had a higher mortality rate, yet most survived at least 1 year after the order. The paradox was that, in the short term, the 'do not resuscitate' order had no impact on measured health-care resource consumption, but for those in the final months of life, in-patient hospital use was less for the 'do not resuscitate' group as most died in the nursing home.

The procedure and process for life-support withdrawal must be considered. Analysis of physician and family end-of-life meetings found that the 'patient's wishes' were a central orientation point for discussion[197]. Physicians tended to provide a direct and unambiguous introduction, giving equal weights to options during decision-framing, but narrowed the options during decision-making to correspond to their own judgements.

The rate of life-support withdrawal was 43% from Kollef's series of 159 MICU patients[198]. He defined three independent predictors associated with support withdrawal, including a planned therapeutic trial of life-sustaining interventions outlined in the medical record, the lack of a private attending physician, and the presence of clearly defined advanced directives regarding patient preferences for medical care. Patients with private attending physicians had significantly greater medical care costs and charges.

The process and outcome of support withdrawal was described in Lee and associates' series of 28 patients with mean APACHE II score of 27.1 ± 7.3 and predicted mortality of $61 \pm 22\%$[199]. The discussion leading to withdrawal of care occurred over 5.2 ± 5.5 days, with the decision to withdraw occurring soonest in cases of poor neurological prognosis. The average MICU stay was only 1.4 ± 1.8 days following the decision to withdraw ICU care, and four patients received more than 48 h of care, while four additional patients were discharged alive from the hospital.

Hence, it appears that families consider outcome when making withdrawal decisions and, interestingly, life-support withdrawal is not uniformly fatal.

Quality of life

Perhaps the most important issue with regard to outcome prediction is quality above length of life. Life certainly becomes more precious as one draws closer to one's demise. Likewise, it is difficult to judge quality of life in a debilitated patient for whom ever-simple pleasures such as enjoying a meal or watching a television show may remain more precious than for the physician.

Patrick and colleagues evaluated 69 patients who underwent MICU care, and found that functional status correlated only moderately with perceived quality of life[200]. Thus, an objectively Perceived Quality-of-Life Scale did not predict satisfaction, mandating the analysis of subjective assessment of patient experience.

Goldstein and co-workers performed a large-scale evaluation of the functional outcome of 2213 MICU and CCU patients based on their premorbid status: sedentary (1017), active (917) or severely limited (279)[201]. Those with severe functional limitation before admission were twice as likely to undergo major interventions, and had higher mortality rates and hospital charges. Hence, overall mortality was 7% for those who were active, 20% for those who were sedentary and 37% for those who were severely impaired. Importantly, 60% of those previously employed were able to return to work after a hospital stay for critical illness.

COST OF CARE

Although thought to be a novel concept, the cost/benefit ratio for MICU care has been a subject of analysis for some time.

Detsky and colleagues evaluated resource expenditure in 1831 MICU and CCU patients, publishing their experience in 1981[202]. The care of non-survivors involved a significantly higher mean financial expenditure than that for survivors, and was greatest for those with unanticipated outcome. The expenditure was positively correlated with probability estimates at time of admission in non-survivors, while it was negatively correlated with survival in those who survived. Hence, prognostic certainty may be a crucial factor in cost analysis.

Franklin and co-workers attempted to clarify triage criteria in 2419 MICU patients, and found considerable overlap in the APACHE physiological score and predicted mortality rate in those admitted[203]. However, there was no discriminate score or mortality rate at which triage criteria would have included most patients who survived without admission to the MICU.

There have been attempts to define extremely low survival-rate groups, to utilize resources better. Chassin evaluated 489 patients who demonstrated an 86% ICU admission and a 72% 6-month survival rate[204]. The average daily ICU cost was $US 1120, with total 6-month charges of $US 14 577 in 1982. The age, initial systolic blood pressure-based preadmission functional status and diagnosis were all independently associated with survival. The subgroup with the lowest 6-month survival of 14% were cancer patients. The practical problem with this approach is that even focusing on this group did not justify withholding of resources to control ICU costs.

The reasons for ICU admission, in addition to age, have been compared with outcome. Fedullo and Swinburne evaluated 182 patients and found the reason for admission to be similar for both older (>70 years) and middle-aged (50–69 years) patients, while only 5% (one of 21) of those with arrest occurring outside of the MICU survived[200]. If cardiac arrest was excluded, then patient survival was 80% in the 5th, 87% in the 6th, 86% in the 7th, 67% in the 8th and 79% in the 9th decade. Some 74% (38 of 51) of the septuagenarian age group were still alive at 6 months, and the costs analyzed from both hospital and ICU stay were similar for both age groups. Thus, age should not be a criterion for resource allocation using this model.

Several studies have addressed the direct influence of insurance status on resource utilization. Mayer-Oakes and colleagues reported the impact of the Medicare prospective payment system (PPS) on 400 patients, 200 pre- and 200 post-institution of the PPS[205]. Comparing Medicare patients (>65 years) with non-Medicare patients (50–65 years), the number of ICU beds decreased by 31% in the Medicare group, while the length of stay decreased by 15% in the Medicare group and 43% in the comparison group. The length of stay decreased by 14% post-PPS, compared to pre-PPS, and patients were less likely to be discharged, but there was no difference in in-hospital or 6-month mortality.

The impact of the diagnosis-related group (DRG) prospective payment on utilization of medical intensive care has been reported as a financial success. Ahmad and associates documented an average cost per discharge of $US 9794 which increased to a $US 11 418 average deficit in the 42% who died in the DRG group, compared to $US 14 113 rising to $US 20 271 for the 39.4% who expired in the medical group, in 1984–85[206]. However, there was no difference in the use of ICU beds after the advent of the DRG method of payment, compared to Medicare.

The importance of the costs of ICU care are illustrated by the 23% ratio of ICU/ward care estimated from Butler and colleagues' analysis of 446 Medicare patients, with a 5-day length of stay in the ICU of the total hospital 22-day stay and an overall 28% mortality rate[207].

Intensive care has been scrutinized as a major factor in increasing health-care costs. Oye and Bellamy examined 404 consecutive admissions for patterns of resource-use consumption[208]. There was a skewed distribution of ICU resources consumption with the 'high-cost' group, constituting 8% of the population, using as many ICU resources as the 'low-cost' patients, constituting 92% of cases. In addition, there were 41% of admissions who did not receive acute ICU treatment, and consumed less than 10% of resources[196,209,210]. Therefore, reducing the number of patients admitted for monitoring will have small impact on hospital charges. Finally, as over 70% of the 'high-cost' patients died, improved understanding of prognosis and better communication may decrease the proportion of critical-care resources expended on futile treatment.

CONCLUSION

The optimum use of ICU resources provides the best care for the majority of patients by aggressive early intervention for all encountered, and rapid decision-making regarding respiratory support. Institution of this potentially life-saving intervention should be based on discussion with the patient and family members, and prognostic estimates to decide the most suitable care, advising on the prospects of meaningful recovery or futility. The ideal decision-making process should maximize patient autonomy in end-of-life decisions ensuring relief of pain and anxiety while maintaining dignity.

REFERENCES

1. Callahan JA, Spiekerman RE, Broadbent JC, *et al*. St. Mary's Hospital–Mayo Clinic Medical Intensive-Care Unit. II. Patient population. *Mayo Clin Proc* 1967;42:332–8

2. Callahan JA, Broadbent JC, Spiekerman RE, *et al.* St. Mary's Hospital–Mayo Clinic medical intensive-care unit. I. *Mayo Clin Proc* 1967;42:326–31

3. Skjaeggestad O, Grendahl H, Hjermann I, *et al.* One year's experience of medical intensive care units. *Acta Med Scand* 1970;187:275–81

4. Spagnolo SV, Hershberg PI, Zimmerman HJ. Medical intensive care unit: mortality rate experience in large teaching hospital. *NY State J Med* 1973;73:754–7

5. Thibault GE, Mulley AG, Barnett GO, *et al.* Medical intensive care: indications, intervention, and outcomes. *N Engl J Med* 1980;302:938–42

6. Eng PC, Chng HH, Feng PH. Mortality patterns in a medical intensive care unit. *Singapore Med J* 1992;33:24–6

7. Staples S. Medical intensive care. *Can Nurs* 1967;63:31–4

8. Clark TJ, Collins JV, Evans TR, *et al.* A review of experience operating a general medical intensive care unit. *Br Med J* 1971;1:158–61

9. Collins JV, Evans TR, Clark TJ. Basic equipment for medical intensive-care units. *Lancet* 1971;1:285–7

10. Mushin WW, Lunn JN. The anaesthetist and intensive care. *Br Med J* 1969;2:683–4

11. Reynolds HN, Haupt MT, Thil-Baharozian MC, *et al.* Impact of critical care physician staffing on patients with septic shock in a university hospital medical intensive care unit. *J Am Med Assoc* 1988;260:3446–50

12. Weiss BD. Family physicians in university hospital intensive care units. *J Fam Pract* 1983;17:683–93

13. Hainer BL, Lawler FH. Comparison of critical care provided by family physicians and general internists. *J Am Med Assoc* 1988;260:354–8

14. Carson SS, Stocking C, Podsadecki T, *et al.* Effects of organizational change in the medical intensive care unit of a teaching hospital: a comparison of 'open' and 'closed' formats. *J Am Med Assoc* 1996;276:322–8

15. Campion EW, Reder VA, Mulley AG, *et al.* Age and the declining rate of autopsy. *J Am Geriatr Soc* 1986;34:865–8

16. Rogers PL, Lane HC, Henderson, DK, *et al.* Admission of AIDS patients to a medical intensive care unit: causes and outcomes. *Crit Care Med* 1989;17:113–17

17. Friedman Y, Franklin C, Freels S, *et al.* Long term survival of patients with AIDS, *Pneumocystis carinii* pneumonia, and respiratory failure. *J Am Med Assoc* 1991;226:89–92

18. Peruzzi WT, Shapiro BA, Noskin GA, *et al.* Concurrent bacterial lung infection in patients with AIDS, PCP, and respiratory failure. *Chest* 1992;101:1399–403

19. Brown MC, Crede WB. Predictive ability of acute physiology and chronic health virus positive patients. *Crit Care Med* 1995;23:848–53

20. McClish DK, Powell SH, Montenegro H, *et al.* The impact of age on utilization of intensive care resources. *J Am Geriat Soc* 1987;35:983–8

21. Campion EW, Mulley AG, Goldstein RL, *et al.* Medical intensive care for the elderly. A study of current use, costs, and outcomes. *J Am Med Assoc* 1981;246:2052–6

22. Wu AW, Rubin HR, Rosen MJ. Are elderly people less responsive to intensive care? *J Am Geriatr Soc* 1990;38:621–7

23. Goldstein RL, Campion EW, Mulley AG, *et al.* Nursing home patients admitted to a medical intensive care unit. *Med Care* 1984;22:854–62

24. Rubins HB, Moskowitz MA. Complications of care in a medical intensive care unit. *J Gen Intern Med* 1990;5:104–9

25. Franklin C, Mathew J. Developing strategies to prevent inhospital cardiac arrest: analyzing responses of physicians and nurses in the hours before the event. *Crit Care Med* 1994;2:244–7

26. Peterson MW, Geist LJ, Schwartz DA, *et al.* Outcome after cardiopulmonary resuscitation in a medical intensive care unit. *Chest* 1991;100: 168–74

27. Silverstein MD, Singer DE, Mulley AG, *et al.* Patients with syncope admitted to medical intensive care units. *J Am Med Assoc* 1982;248:1185–9

28. Mulley AG, Thibault GE, Hughes RA, *et al.* The course of patients with suspected myocardial infarction. *N Engl J Med* 1980;302:943–8

29. Gulsvik A, Hansteen V, Sivertssen E. Cardiac arrhythmias in patients with serious pulmonary diseases. *Scand J Resp Dis* 1978;59:154–9

30. Fernandes A, Santos JM, Lima JV, *et al.* Unstable angina. An evaluation of a diagnostic and therapeutic methodology. *Rev Portuguesa Cardiol* 1993;12:1023–7

31. Ludwigs U, Hulting J. Acute physiology and chronic health evaluation II scoring system in acute myocardial infarction: a prospective validation study. *Crit Care Med* 1995;23:854–9

32. Mulcahy D, Fitzgerald M, Wright C, *et al.* Long term follow up of severely ill patients who underwent urgent cardiac transplantation. *Br Med J* 1993;306:98–101

33. Wiener F, Weil MH. Cardiovascular monitoring in the medical intensive care unit. *Med Instrum* 1977;11:268–73

34. Alcover IA, Henning RJ, Jackson DL. A computer assisted monitoring system for arrhythmia detection in a medical intensive care unit. *Crit Care Med* 1984;12:888–91

35. Jain P, Parada JP, David A, *et al.* Overuse of the indwelling urinary tract catheter in hospitalized medical patients. *Arch Intern Med* 1995;155:1425–9

36. Roos AN, Westendorp RG, Frolich M, *et al.* Weight changes in critically ill patients evaluated by fluid balances and impedance measurements. *Crit Care Med* 1993;21:871–7

37. Dale JC, Pruett SK. Phlebotomy – a minimalist approach. *Mayo Clin Proc* 1993;68:249–55

38. Venkatesh B, Clutton Brock TH, Hendry SP. A multiparameter sensor for continuous intra-arterial blood gas monitoring: a prospective evaluation. *Crit Care Med* 1994;22:588–94

39. Zimmerman JL, Dellinger RP. Initial evaluation of a new intra-arterial blood gas system in humans. *Crit Care Med* 1993;21:495–500

40. Silver MJ, Li YH, Gragg LA, *et al*. Reduction of blood loss from diagnostic sampling in critically ill patients using a blood conserving arterial line system. *Chest* 1993;104:1711–15

41. Peruzzi WT, Parker MA, Lichtenthal PR, *et al*. A clinical evaluation of a blood conservation device in medical intensive care unit patients. *Crit Care Med* 1993;21:501–6

42. Ganz W, Donoso R, Marcus HS, *et al*. A new technique for measurement of cardiac output by thermodilution in man. *Am J Cardiol* 1970; 27:392–6

43. Branthwaite MA, Bradley RD. Measurement of cardiac output by thermal dilution in man. *J Appl Physiol* 1968;24:434–8

44. Sasse SA, Chen PA, Berry RB, *et al*. Variability of cardiac output over time in medical intensive care unit patients. *Crit Care Med* 1994;22:225–32

45. Unger KM, Shibel EM, Moser KM. Detection of left ventricular failure in patients with adult respiratory distress syndrome. *Chest* 1975;67:8–13

46. Mimoz O, Rauss A, Rekik N, *et al*. Pulmonary artery catheterization in critically ill patients. A prospective analysis of outcome changes associated with catheter-prompted changes in therapy. *Crit Care Med* 1994;22:573–9

47. Coles NA, Hibberd M, Russell M, *et al*. Potential impact of pulmonary artery catheter placement on short term management decisions in the medical intensive care unit. *Am Heart J* 1993;126:815–19

48. Plit ML, Rumbak MJ, Lipman J, *et al*. Invasive vascular catheterization in the critically ill. *S Afr Med J* 1987;72:245–8

49. Morris D, Mulvihill D, Lew WY. Risk of developing complete heart block during bedside pulmonary artery catheterization in patients with left bundle-branch block. *Arch Intern Med* 1987;147:2005–10

50. Fahey PJ, Harris K, Vanderwarf C. Clinical experience with continuous monitoring of mixed venous oxygen saturation in respiratory failure. *Chest* 1984;86:748–52

51. Kreymann G, Grosser S, Buggisch P, *et al*. Oxygen consumption and resting metabolic rate in sepsis, sepsis syndrome, and septic shock. *Crit Care Med* 1993;21:1012–19

52. Vukmir RB, Darby J, Peitzman A, *et al.* End diastolic volume: correlation with cardiac output in blunt thoracic trauma patients. *Crit Care Med* 1994;22:A72

53. Roos AN, Westendorp RG, Brand R, *et al.* Predictive value of tetrapolar body impedance measurements for hydration status in critically ill patients. *Intens Care Med* 1995;21:125–31

54. Connors AF Jr, Speroff T, Dawson NV. The effectiveness of right heart catheterization in the initial care of critically ill patients. *J Am Med Assoc* 1996;276:889–97

55. Goeckenjan G, Seidel R, Trampisch HJ, *et al.* Acute respiratory failure in a medical intensive care unit. *Deutsche Med Wochenschr* 1984;109:563–8

56. Swinburne AJ, Fedullo AJ, Bixby K, *et al.* Respiratory failure in the elderly. Analysis of outcome after treatment with mechanical ventilation. *Arch Intern Med* 1993;153:1657–62

57. Papadakis MA, Lee KK, Browner WS, *et al.* Prognosis of mechanically ventilated patients. *West J Med* 1993;159:659–64

58. Ludwigs UG, Baehrendtz S, Wanecek M, *et al.* Mechanical ventilation in medical and neurological diseases: 11 years of experience. *J Intern Med* 1991;229:117–24

59. Braman SS, Kaemmerlen JT. Intensive care of status asthmaticus: a 10 year experience. *J Am Med Assoc* 1990;264:366–8

60. Pacht ER, Lingo S, St John RC. Clinical features, management, and outcome of patients with severe asthma admitted to the intensive care unit. *J Asthma* 1995;32:373–87

61. Lim TK. Status asthmaticus in medical intensive care. *Singapore Med J* 1989;30:334–8

62. Bartter T, Pratter MR. Asthma: better outcome at lower cost? The role of the expert in the care system. *Chest* 1996;110:1589–96

63. Dahmash NS, Chowdhury MN. Re-evaluation of pneumonia requiring admission to an intensive care unit: a prospective study. *Thorax* 1994;49:71–6

64. Limthongkul S, Charoenlap P. Community and hospital acquired pneumonia in medical intensive care unit. *J Med Assoc Thailand* 1993;76:129–37

65. Norwood SH, Civetta JM. Ventilatory support in patients with ARDS. *Surg Clin North Am* 1985;65:895–916

66. Gammon RB, Shin MS, Buchalter SE. Pulmonary barotrauma in mechanical ventilation, patterns and risk factors. *Chest* 1992;102:568–72

67. Lain DC, Di Benedetto R, Nguyen AV, *et al.* Pressure control inverse ratio ventilation as a method to reduce peak inspiratory pressure and provide adequate ventilation and oxygenation. *Chest* 1989;95:1081–8

68. Moalli R, Doyle JM, Tahhan HR, *et al.* Fibrinolysis in critically ill patients. *Am Rev Resp Dis* 1989;140:287–93
69. Dahmash NS, Arora SC, Fayed DF. Infection in critically ill patients: experience in MICU at a major teaching hospital. *Infection* 1994; 22:264–70
70. Craven DE, Kunches LM, Lichtenberg DA, *et al.* Nosocomial infection and fatality in medical and surgical intensive care unit patients. *Arch Intern Med* 1988;148:1161–8
71. Bauer TM, Ofner E, Just HM, *et al.* An epidemiological study assessing the relative importance of airborne and direct contact transmission of microorganisms in a medical intensive care unit. *J Hosp Infect* 1990; 15:301–9
72. Rose HD, Babcock JB. Colonization of intensive care unit patients with gram-negative bacilli. *Am J Epidemiol* 1975;101:495–501
73. Weinstein JW, Roe M, Towns M, *et al.* Resistant enterococci: a prospective study of prevalence, incidence, and factors associated with colonization in a university hospital. *Infect Control Hosp Epidemiol* 1996;17:36–41
74. Frame RN, Johnson MC, Eichenhorn MS, *et al.* Active tuberculosis in the medical intensive care unit: a 15 year retrospective analysis. *Crit Care Med* 1987;15:1012–14
75. Griffith DE, Hardeman JL, Zhang Y, *et al.* Tuberculosis outbreak among healthcare workers in a community hospital. *Am J Resp Crit Care Med* 1995;152:808–11
76. Henderson DK, Baptiste R, Parrillo J, *et al.* Indolent epidemic of *Pseudomonas cepacia* bacteremia and pseudobacteremia in an intensive care unit traced to a contaminated blood gas analyzer. *Am J Med* 1988; 84:75–81
77. Cortes JL, Cominguez-de Villota E, Algora-Weber A, *et al.* Sequential epidemic outbreaks of septicaemias by *Serratia* and *Klebsiella* species on a medical intensive care unit. *Intens Care Med* 1988;14:126–40
78. Rimailho A, Lampl E, Riou B, *et al.* Enterococcal bacteremia in a medical intensive care unit. *Crit Care Med* 1988;16:126–9
79. Crossley KB, Ross J. Colonization of hospitalized patients by *Staphylococcus aureus, Staphylococcus epidermidis,* and enterococci. *J Hosp Infect* 1985;6:179–86
80. Vazquez JA, Sanchez V, Dmuchowski C, *et al.* Nosocomial acquisition of *Candida albicans*: an epidemiologic study. *J Infect Dis* 1993;168: 195–201
81. Guidry GG, Black-Payne CA, Payne DK, *et al.* Respiratory syncytial virus infection among intubated adults in a university medical intensive care unit. *Chest* 1991;100:1377–84

82. Slaughter S, Hayden MK, Nathan C, *et al*. A comparison of the effect of universal use of gloves and gowns with that of glove use alone on acquisition of vancomycin-resistant enterococci in a medical intensive care unit. *Ann Int Med* 1996;125:448–56

83. Kotilainen HR, Brinker JP, Avato JL, *et al*. Latex and vinyl examination gloves, quality control procedures and implications for health care workers. *Arch Intern Med* 1989;149:2749–53

84. Ullman RF, Gurevich I, Schoch PE, *et al*. Colonization and bacteremia related to duration of triple-lumen intravascular catheter placement. *Am J Infect Control* 1990;18:201–7

85. Dominguez de Villota E, Algora A, Rubio JJ, *et al*. Septicaemia in a medical intensive care unit. *Intens Care Med* 1983;9:109–15

86. Gross PA, Van Antwerpen CL, Hess WA, *et al*. Use and abuse of blood cultures: program to limit use. *Am J Infect Control* 1988;16:114–17

87. Baumgartner JD, Bula C, Vaney C, *et al*. A novel score for predicting the mortality of septic shock patients. *Crit Care Med* 1992;20:953–60

88. Knothe H. Antibiotic usage for initial empirical treatment of infections in hospitalized patients in West Germany. *Infection* 1991;19:127–30

89. Ben-Menachem T, Fogel R, Patel RV, *et al*. Prophylaxis for stress-related gastric hemorrhage in the medical intensive care unit. A randomized, controlled single-blind study. *Ann Int Med* 1994;121:568–75

90. Schuster DP, Rowley H, Feinstein S, *et al*. Prospective evaluation of the risk of upper gastrointestinal bleeding after admission to a medical intensive care unit. *Am J Med* 1984;76:623–30

91. Kollef MH, Canfield DA, Zuckerman GR. Triage considerations for patients with acute gastrointestinal hemorrhage admitted to a medical intensive care unit. *Crit Care Med* 1995;23:1048–54

92. Deus JR, Marques A, Santos P, *et al*. Acute pancreatitis, inflammatory effusions, course and prognosis. *Acta Med Portuguesa* 1989;2:189–94

93. National Center Health Statistics. *Vital statistics of the United States.* DHHS Publications no. (PHS) 88–11222. Hyattsville, Maryland: US Department of Health and Human Services, 1986

94. Turcotte JG, Child CG. Portal hypertension: pathogenesis, management, and prognosis. *Post Grad Med* 1967;41:93–101

95. Shellman RG, Fulkerson WJ, DeLong E, *et al*. Prognosis of patients with cirrhosis and chronic liver disease admitted to the medical intensive care unit. *Crit Care Med* 1988;16:671–8

96. Groeneveld AB, Tran DD, van der Meulen J, *et al*. Acute renal failure in the medical intensive care unit: predisposing, complicating factors and outcome. *Nephron* 1991;59:602–10

97. Schaefer JH, Jochimsen F, Keller F, *et al.* Outcome prediction of acute renal failure in medical intensive care. *Intens Care Med* 1991; 17:19–24

98. Jochimsen F, Schafer JH, Maurer A, *et al.* Impairment of renal function in medical intensive care: predictability of acute renal failure. *Crit Care Med* 1990;18:480–5

99. Druml W, Lax F, Grimm G, *et al.* Acute renal failure in the elderly 1975–1990. *Clin Nephrol* 1994;41:342–9

100. Tasseau F, Gaucher L, Nicolas F. Cell-mediated immunity studied by skin tests in patients receiving intensive care. Prognostic value of repeated tests. Study of some factors predisposing towards anergy [in French]. *Semaine Hop* 1982;58:781–4

101. Pixley RA, Zellis S, Bankes P, *et al.* Prognostic value of assessing contact system activation and factor V in systemic inflammatory response syndrome. *Crit Care Med* 1995;23:41–51

102. Arnalich F, Sanchez JF, Martinez M, *et al.* Changes in plasma concentrations of vasoactive neuropeptides in patients with sepsis and septic shock. *Life Sci* 1995;56:75–81

103. Zeni F, Pain P, Vindimian M, *et al.* Effects of pentoxifylline on circulating cytokine concentrations and hemodynamics in patients with septic shock: results from a double-blind, randomized, placebo-controlled study. *Crit Care Med* 1996;24:207–14

104. Casey LC, Balk RA, Bone RC. Plasma cytokine and endotoxin levels correlate with survival in patients with the sepsis syndrome. *Ann Int Med* 1993;119:771–8

105. Friedland JS, Porter JC, Daryanani S, *et al.* Plasma proinflammatory cytokine concentrations, Acute Physiology and Chronic Health Evaluation (APACHE) III scores and survival in patients in an intensive care unit. *Crit Care Med* 1996;24:1775–81

106. Offner F, Philipee J, Vogelaers D, *et al.* Serum tumor necrosis factor levels in patients with infectious disease and septic shock. *J Lab Clin Med* 1990;116:100–5

107. Lin RY, Astiz ME, Saxon JC, *et al.* Relationships between plasma cytokine concentrations and leukocyte functional antigen expression in patients with sepsis. *Crit Care Med* 1994;22:1595–602

108. Lee KH, Hui KP, Tan WC. Thrombocytopenia in sepsis: a predictor of mortality in the intensive care unit. *Singapore Med J* 1993;34: 245–6

109. Schuster DP, Marion JM. Precedents for meaningful recovery during treatment in a medical intensive care unit. Outcome in patients with hematologic malignancy. *Am J Med* 1983;75:402–8

110. Brunet F, Lanore JJ, Dhainaut JF, *et al.* Is intensive care justified for patients with haematological malignancies? *Intens Care Med* 1990; 16:291–7

111. Ashkenazi YJ, Kramer BS, Harman E. Short-term outcome among patients with leukemia and lymphoma admitted to a medical intensive care unit. *South Med J* 1986;79:1086–8

112. Paz HL, Crilley P, Weinar M, *et al.* Outcome of patients requiring medical ICU admission following bone marrow transplantation. *Chest* 1993;104:527–31

113. Papadakis MA, Mangione CM, Lee KK, *et al.* Treatable abdominal pathologic conditions and unsuspected malignant neoplasms at autopsy in veterans who received mechanical ventilation. *J Am Med Assoc* 1991;265:885–7

114. Sculier JP, Markiewicz E. Medical cancer patients and intensive care. *Anticancer Res* 1991;11:2172–4

115. Sculier JP, Markiewicz E. Cardiopulmonary resuscitation in medical cancer patients: the experience of a medical intensive care unit of a cancer center. *Support Care Cancer* 1993;1:135–8

116. Strain DS, Kinasewitz GT, Vereen LE, *et al.* Value of routine daily chest X-rays in the medical intensive care unit. *Crit Care Med* 1985;13:534–6

117. Henschke CI, Pasternack GS, Schroeder S, *et al.* Bedside chest radiography: diagnostic efficacy. *Radiology* 1983;149:23–6

118. Greenbaum DM, Marshcall KE. The value of routine daily chest X-rays in intubated patients in the medical intensive care unit. *Crit Care Med* 1982;10:29–30

119. Boles JM, Boussert F, Manens JP, *et al.* Measurement of irradiation doses secondary to bedside radiographs in a medical intensive care unit. *Intens Care Med* 1987;13:60–3

120. Arenson RL, Seshadri SB, Kundel HL, *et al.* Clinical evaluation of a medical image management system for chest images. *Am J Roentgenol* 1988;150:55–9

121. Tucker DM, McEachern M. Quality assurance and quality control of an intensive care unit picture archiving and communication system. *J Dig Imag* 1995;8:162–7

122. Szalados JE, Vukmir RB. Acute adrenal insufficiency resulting from adrenal hemorrhage as indicated by post-operative hypotension. *Intens Care Med* 1994;20:216–18

123. Bouachour G, Tirot P, Gouello JP, *et al.* Adrenocortical function during septic shock. *Intens Care Med* 1995;21:57–62

124. Lelarge P, Bollaert PE, Bauer P, *et al.* Treatment of severe hyponatremia by restricted water intake [in French]. *Presse Med* 1989;18:517–20

125. Davenport MW, Zipser RD. Association of hypotension with hypo-reninemic hypoaldosteronism in the critically ill patient. *Arch Intern Med* 1983;143:735–7

126. Melmed S, Geola RL, Reed AW, *et al.* A comparison of methods for assessing thyroid function in nonthyroidal illness. *J Clin Endocrinol Metab* 1982;54:300–6

127. Desai TK, Carlson RW, Geheb MA. Prevalence and clinical implications of hypocalcemia in acutely ill patients in a medical intensive care setting. *Am J Med* 1988;84:209–14

128. Hirsch DR, Ingenito EP, Goldhaber SZ. Prevalence of deep venous thrombosis among patients in medical intensive care. *J Am Med Assoc* 1995;274:335–7

129. Habscheid W, Stratmann A, Dammrich J. KompressionSonographie als Screening Method in der Thrombosediagnostik. *Deutsche Med Wochenschr* 1990;115:1003–8

130. Keane MG, Ingenito EP, Goldhaber SZ. Utilization of venous thromboembolism prophylaxis in the medical intensive care unit. *Chest* 1994;106:13–14

131. Godeau B, Boudjadja A, Dhainaut JF, *et al.* Outcome of patients with systemic rheumatic disease admitted to medical intensive care units. *Ann Rheum Dis* 1992;51:627–31

132. Muller TF, Muller A, Bachem MG, *et al.* Immediate metabolic effects of different nutritional regimens in critically ill medical patients. *Intens Care Med* 1995;21:561–6

133. Larca L, Greenbaum DM. Effectiveness of intensive nutritional regimes in patients who fail to wean from mechanical ventilation. *Crit Care Med* 1982;10:297–300

134. Abramson NS, Safar P, Detre KM, *et al.* Neurologic recovery after cardiac arrest: effect of duration of ischemia. *Crit Care Med* 1985;13:930–1

135. Levy DE, Caronna JJ, Singer BH. Predicting outcome from hypoxic–ischemic coma. *J Am Med Assoc* 1985;253:1420–6

136. van der Hoeven JG, de Koning J, Compier EA, *et al.* Early jugular bulb oxygenation monitoring in comatose patients after an out-of-hospital cardiac arrest. *Intens Care Med* 1995;21:567–72

137. Madl C, Kramer L, Yeganehfar W, *et al.* Detection of nontraumatic comatose patients with no benefit of intensive care treatment by recording of sensory evoked potentials. *Arch Neurol* 1996;53:512–16

138. Hund EF, Fogel W, Krieger D, *et al.* Critical illness polyneuropathy: clinical findings and outcomes of a frequent cause of neuromuscular weaning failure. *Crit Care Med* 1996;24:1328–33

139. Kathol RG, Henn FA. Tricyclics, the most common agent used in potentially lethal overdoses. *J Nerv Ment Dis* 1983;171:250–2

140. Sloth-Madsen P, Strom J, Reiz S, *et al.* Acute propoxyphene self-poisoning in 222 consecutive patients. *Acta Anaesth Scand* 1984;28:661–5

141. Kallenbach J, Bagg P, Feldman C, *et al.* Experience with acute poisoning in an intensive care unit. A review of 103 cases. *S Afr Med J* 1981;59:587–9

142. Heyman EN, LoCastro DE, Gouse LH, *et al.* Intentional drug overdose: predictors of clinical course in the intensive care unit. *Heart Lung* 1996;25:246–52

143. Stern TA, Mulley AG, Thibault GE. Life threatening drug overdose, precipitants and prognosis. *J Am Med Assoc* 1984;251:1983–5

144. Ojehagen A, Danielsson M, Traskman-Bendz L. Deliberate self-poisoning: treatment follow up of repeaters and nonrepeaters. *Acta Psychiatr Scand* 1992;85:370–5

145. Baldwin WA, Rosenfeld BA, Breslow MJ, *et al.* Substance abuse related admissions to adult intensive care. *Chest* 1993;103:21–5

146. Smythe MA, Melendy S, Jahns B, *et al.* An exploratory analysis of medication utilization in a medical intensive care unit. *Crit Care Med* 1993;21:1319–23

147. Dager WE, Albertson TE. Impact of therapeutic drug monitoring of intravenous theophylline regimens on serum theophylline concentrations in the medical intensive care unit. *Ann Pharmacother* 1992;26:1287–91

148. Katona BG, Ayd PR, Walters JK, *et al.* Effect of a pharmacist's and a nurse's interventions on cost of drug therapy in a medical intensive care unit. *Am J Hosp Pharm* 1989;46:1179–82

149. Smego RA, Durack DT. The neuroleptic malignant syndrome. *Arch Intern Med* 1982;142:1183–5

150. Whitcup SM, Miller F. Unrecognized drug dependence in psychiatrically hospitalized elderly patients. *J Am Geriatr Soc* 1987;35:297–301

151. Scherubel JC, Tess MM. Measuring clinical confusion in critically ill patients. *J Neurosci Nurs* 1994;26:146–50

152. Schilling G, Scheer JW, Laubach W, *et al.* Psychopathology, coping and defence in intensive care patients. *Fortschr Neurol Psychiatrie* 1994;62:233–40

153. Edwards GB, Schuring LM. Pilot study: validating staff nurses' observations of sleep and wake states among critically ill patients, using polysomnography. *Am J Crit Care* 1993;2:125–31

154. Cray L. A collaborative project: initiating a family intervention program in a medical intensive care unit. *Focus Crit Care* 1989;16:213–18

155. Perez-San Gregorio MA, Blanco-Picabia A, Murillo-Cabezas F, *et al.* Psychological problems in the family members of gravely traumatized patients admitted into an intensive care unit. *Intens Care Med* 1992;18:278–81

156. Henneman EA, McKenzie JB, Dewa CS. An evaluation of interventions for meeting the information needs of families of critically ill patients. *Am J Crit Care* 1992;1:85–93

157. Lerch MM, Riehl J, Buechsel R, *et al.* Bedside ultrasound in decision making for emergency surgery: its role in medical intensive care patients. *Am J Emerg Med* 1992;10:35–8

158. Kollef MH, Allen BT. Determinants of outcome for patients in the medical intensive care unit requiring abdominal surgery: a prospective, single-center study. *Chest* 1994;106:1822–8

159. Kirshon B, Hinkley CM, Cotton DB, *et al.* Maternal mortality in a maternal fetal medicine intensive care unit. *J Reprod Med* 1990;35:25–8

160. Collop NA, Sahn SA. Critical illness in pregnancy: an analysis of 20 patients admitted to a medical intensive care unit. *Chest* 1993;103: 1548–52

161. Sivak ED, Perez-Trepichio A. Quality assessment in the medical intensive care unit: evolution of a data model [published erratum appears in *Cleve Clin J Med* 1990;57:654]. *Cleve Clin J Med* 1990;57:273–9

162. Sivak ED, Perez-Trepichio A. Quality assessment in the medical intensive care unit. *Qual Assur Utiliz Rev* 1992;7:42–9

163. Donabedian A. The quality of care, how can it be assessed? *J Am Med Assoc* 1988;260:1743–8

164. Kruse JA, Thill-Baharozian MC, Carlson RW. Comparison of clinical assessment with APACHE II for predicting mortality risk in patients admitted to a medical intensive care unit. *J Am Med Assoc* 1988; 260:1739–42

165. Schafer JH, Maurer A, Jochimsen F, *et al.* Outcome prediction models on admission in a medical intensive care unit: do they predict individual outcome? *Crit Care Med* 1990;18:1111–18

166. Gross PA, Stein MR, van Antwerpen C, *et al.* Comparison of severity of illness indicators in an intensive care unit. *Arch Intern Med* 1991;151:2201–5

167. Brown PE, McClave SA, Hoy NW, *et al.* The acute physiology and chronic health evaluation II classification system is a valid marker for physiologic stress in the critically ill patient. *Crit Care Med* 1993; 21:363–7

168. Tran DD, Groeneveld AB, van der Meulen J, *et al.* Age, chronic disease, sepsis, organ system failure, and mortality in a medical intensive care unit. *Crit Care Med* 1990;18:474–9

169. Kollef MH. The identification of ICU-specific outcome predictors: a comparison of medical, surgical, and cardiothoracic ICUs from a single institution. *Heart Lung* 1995;24:60–6

170. Escarce JJ, Kelley MA. Admission source to the medical intensive care unit predicts hospital death independent of APACHE II score. *J Am Med Assoc* 1990;264:2389–94

171. Lee KH, Hui KP, Lim TK, *et al.* Acute physiology and chronic health evaluation (APACHE II) scoring in the Medical Intensive Care Unit, National University Hospital, Singapore. *Singapore Med J* 1993;34:41–4

172. Brannen AL, Godfrey LG, Goetter WE. Prediction of outcome from critical illness. A comparison of clinical judgement with a prediction rule. *Arch Intern Med* 1989;149:1083–6

173. Christensen C, Cottrell JJ, Murakami J, *et al.* Forecasting survival in the medical intensive care unit: a comparison of clinical prognoses with formal estimates. *Meth Inf Med* 1993;32:302–8

174. Youngner S, Jackson DL, Allen M. Staff attitudes towards the care of the critically ill in the medical intensive care unit. *Crit Care Med* 1979; 7:35–40

175. Cochran LL, Ambutas SA, Buckley JK, *et al.* The unification model: a collaborative effort. *Nurs Conn* 1989;2:5–17

176. Van Buskirk MC, Vanderbilt D. Evaluating patient care by the use of diabetic ketoacidosis care map in an intensive care setting. *J Nurs Care Qual* 1995;9:59–68

177. Baggs JG, Ryan SA, Phelps CE, *et al.* The association between interdisciplinary collaboration and patient outcomes in a medical intensive care unit. *Heart Lung* 1992;21:18–24

178. Cullen DJ, Civetta JM, Briggs BA, *et al.* Therapeutic intervention scoring system: a method for quantitative comparison of patient care. *Crit Care Med* 1974;2:57–60

179. Adam BA, Kin LC, Wahab AS. Therapeutic intervention scoring system in medical intensive care. *Med J Malaysia* 1989;44:134–9

180. Thorens JB, Kaelin RM, Jolliet P, *et al.* Influence of the quality of nursing on the duration of weaning from mechanical ventilation in patients with chronic obstructive pulmonary disease. *Crit Care Med* 1995;23:1807–15

181. Fok AC, Tan YT, Ong YY. Medical intensive care unit utilization in an acute teaching hospital. *Singapore Med J* 1992;33:21–3

182. Kelley MA, Nachamkin DC, Escarce JJ, *et al.* Expansion of the medical intensive care unit: clinical consequences in a large urban hospital. *Crit Care Med* 1990;18:945–9

183. Bone RC, McElwee NE, Eubanks DH, *et al.* Analysis of indications for intensive care unit admission, clinical efficacy assessment project: American College of Physicians. *Chest* 1993;104:1806–11

184. Rubins HB, Moskowitz MA. Discharge decision-making in a medical intensive care unit. Identifying patients at high risk of unexpected death or unit readmission. *Am J Med* 1988;84:863–9

185. Eagle KA, Mulley AG, Skates SJ, *et al.* Length of stay in the intensive care unit. Effects of practice guidelines and feedback. *J Am Med Assoc* 1990;264:992–7

186. Bone RC, McElwee NE, Eubanks DH, *et al.* Analysis of indications for early discharge from the intensive care unit, clinical efficacy assessment project: American College of Physicians. *Chest* 1993;104:1812–17

187. Estrada CA, Rosman HS, Prasad NK, *et al.* Role of telemetry monitoring in the non-intensive care unit. *Am J Cardiol* 1995;76:960–5

188. Elpern EH, Silver MR, Rosen RL, *et al.* The noninvasive respiratory care unit, patterns of use and financial implications. *Chest* 1991; 99:205–8

189. Zimmerman JE, Wagner DP, Knaus WA, *et al.* The use of risk predictions to identify candidates for intermediate care units, implications for intensive care utilization and cost. *Chest* 1995; 108:490–9

190. Byrick RJ, Mazer D, Caskennette GM. Closure of an intermediate care unit, impact on critical care utilization. *Chest* 1993;104:876–81

191. Danis M, Patrick DL, Southerland LI, *et al.* Patients' and families' preferences for medical intensive care. *J Am Med Assoc* 1988;260:797–802

192. Johnson RF Jr, Baranowski-Birkmeier T, O'Donnell JB. Advance directives in the medical intensive care unit of a community teaching hospital. *Chest* 1995;107:752–6

193. Blackhall LJ, Cobb J, Moskowitz MA. Discussions regarding aggressive care with critically ill patients. *J Gen Intern Med* 1989;4:399–402

194. Youngner SJ, Lewandowski W, McClish DK, *et al.* 'Do not resuscitate' orders: incidence and implications in a medical intensive care unit. *J Am Med Assoc* 1985;253:54–7

195. Halevy A, Neal RC, Brody BA. The low frequency of futility in an adult intensive care unit setting. *Arch Intern Med* 1996;156:100–4

196. Kellogg FR, Ramos A. Code status and decision making in a nursing home population: processes and outcomes. *J Am Geriatr Soc* 1995;43: 113–21

197. Miller DK, Coe RM, Hyers TM. Achieving consensus on withdrawing or withholding care for critically ill patients. *J Gen Intern Med* 1992;7: 475–80
198. Kollef MH. Private attending physician status and the withdrawal of life-sustaining interventions in a medical intensive care unit population. *Crit Care Med* 1996;24:968–75
199. Lee DK, Swinburne AJ, Fedullo AJ, *et al.* Withdrawing care. Experience in a medical intensive care unit. *J Am Med Assoc* 1994;271:1358–61
200. Patrick DL, Danis M, Southerland LI, *et al.* Relationship of patient age to cost and survival in a medical ICU. *Crit Care Med* 1983;11:155–9
201. Goldstein RL, Campion EW, Thibault GE, *et al.* Functional outcomes following medical intensive care. *Crit Care Med* 1986;14:783–8
202. Detsky AS, Stricker SC, Mulley AG, *et al.* Prognosis, survival, and the expenditure of hospital resources for patients in an intensive-care unit. *N Engl J Med* 1981;305:667–72
203. Franklin C, Rackow EC, Madamni B, *et al.* Triage considerations in medical intensive care. *Arch Intern Med* 1990;150:1455–9
204. Chassin MR. Costs and outcomes of medical intensive care. *Med Care* 1982;20:165–79
205. Mayer-Oakes SA, Oye RK, Leake B, *et al.* The early effect of Medicare's prospective payment system on the use of medical intensive care services in three community hospitals. *J Am Med Assoc* 1988;260:3146–9
206. Ahmad M, Fergus L, Stothard P, *et al.* Impact of diagnosis-related groups prospective payment on utilization of medical intensive care. *Chest* 1988;93:176–9
207. Butler PW, Bone RC, Field T. Technology under Medicare diagnosis-related groups prospective payment: implications for medical intensive care. *Chest* 1985;87:229–34
208. Oye RK, Bellamy PE. Patterns of resource consumption in medical intensive care. *Chest* 1991;99:685–9
209. Brown MC, Crede WB. Predictive ability of acute physiology and chronic health virus-positive patients. *Crit Care Med* 1995;23:848–53
210. Adams J, Franklin C. Prognosis of patients with cirrhosis and chronic liver diseases admitted to the medical intensive care unit. *Crit Care Med* 1989;17:843–4

2
Perioperative assessment, care and outcome of the critically ill patient

INTRODUCTION

The care of the acutely ill surgical patient begins in the preoperative period and extends through intensive care and the recovery period.

Admission to a surgical intensive care unit (SICU) system is warranted for patients with poor preoperative condition, extensive surgery, significant complications or severe trauma[1]. The internist often assists the operating team in managing the patient's perioperative course in disease states such as malignancy[2]. This practice appears to be more common in private community hospital intensive care units. Trask and Faber's pooled data from 188 facilities[3] suggest that the operating surgeon assumes the primary role in postoperative management in only 20–25% of cases. The rationale for this position includes a rapidly advancing body of critical care knowledge and technology, lack of economic incentive and professional liability concern[3].

The goal of intervention is to provide a multidisciplinary care approach[1]. This strategy, discussed by Frey[4], unites the approaches of the internist who assesses, optimizes function and minimizes impairment of organ systems; the anesthetist who assesses operative risk and attempts acute physiological correction; and the surgeon who provides definitive intervention. The multidisciplinary critical care specialist may support the common therapeutic end-point by closely monitoring perioperative diagnosis and intervention.

ANESTHESIA

There has been significant improvement in outcome from operative intervention, demonstrated by a four-fold reduction in mortality from 1:2680 in 1950 to 1:10 000 in 1985, cited by Davies and Strunin[5]. Anesthetic mortality is more likely to be a result of human error, drug overdose, coexistent disease or failure of postoperative care, rather

77

than equipment failure, poor preoperative assessment or hepatitis caused by inhalational agents or malignant hyperthermia[5]. Perhaps the greatest anesthesia concern is an intraoperative myocardial infarction. Wylie's analysis of 66 anesthetic deaths[6] suggests that 50% of intra-operative cardiac arrests are preventable, with 18% potentially inter-preted as negligence with anesthesia liability for events occurring in the preoperative assessment or postoperative care phases.

The preoperative anesthesia grading scale allows a qualitative assessment of the patient's operative risk (Table 1)[7–12]. Saklad[7] developed a four-stage system with an auxiliary emergency qualifier, comparing physical state and operative risk. The first anesthesia grading system validation developed by Dripps and colleagues[8] examined 33 224 patients and demonstrated 0% intraoperative mortality in the 16 000 healthy patients, while as many as 10% of those with life-threatening illness may have succumbed during general anesthesia. The American Society of Anesthesiologists[9] published a descriptive classification of physical status consisting of five groups with an emergency modifier. The most widely used version is the Goldman multifactorial index of cardiac risk, a qualitative scale that concentrates on cardiac dysfunction as the most significant cause of perioperative morbidity and mortality, based on a 1001-patient group[10]. Zeldin and Math[11] successfully validated this model in 1140 patients who underwent non-cardiac surgical proce-dures. Detsky and co-workers' revised multifactorial index of cardiac risk[12] again stressed the importance of both acute and chronic myo-cardial dysfunction, reported as the likelihood ratio of complications during minor or major surgical intervention in a 455-patient group.

A preoperative assessment is imperative to detect subsequent anesthesia-related complications. This evaluation resulted in delay of operative intervention in 11% of cases owing to requests for physical therapy (6%), hypertension control (4%) or presence of myocardial infarction (1%) in 100 patients studied by Holdcroft[13]. Preoperative laboratory assessment, although routinely performed, is questionable as a screening tool. Screening laboratory testing in 86 healthy, elective orthopedic surgery patients resulted in cancellation of surgery in only 4% of cases owing to the presence of abnormalities upon urinalysis (3%) or liver function testing (1%), based on an evaluation by Sanders and colleagues[14]. Postoperative complications were not predicted by testing (0%), although bleeding was encountered in a patient with hepatitis, despite normal liver function and coagulation tests[14].

78

Table 1 Anesthesia and surgical mortality. Data from references 7–12

System	Complications (%)	Grading				
		I	II	III	IV	V
Saklad 1941		normal or localized disease	moderate systemic	severe systemic	life-threatening	emergency
Dripps *et al.*, 1961	minor	100	97	93	78	
	major	0	2	4	17	
	mortality	0	1	2	5	
American Society of Anesthesiologists, 1963: classification of physical status		Normal healthy	mild systemic	severe systemic	incapacitating systemic	moribund
Goldman *et al.*, 1977: multifactorial index of cardiac risk*		0–5	6–12	13–25	26–53	
	minor	99	93	86	22	
	major	0.7	5	11	22	
	mortality	0.2	2	2	56	
Zeldin and Math, 1984	minor	99	97	85	70	
	major	0.5	2	11	14	
	mortality	0.2	1	4	26	

Table 1   Continued over

Table 1 *Continued*

System	Complications (%)		Grading				
		I	II	III	IV	V
		0–15	15–30	>30		
Detsky et al., 1986:						
revised cardiac	minor surgery	0.4	2.7	12.2		
multifactorial	major surgery	0.4	3.6	14.9		
index†	total	0.4	3.4	10.6		
Cumulative	minor	99	96	88	51	
	major	0.4	3.0	8.7	18	
	mortality	0.1	1.3	2.7	29	

*History: myocardial infarction <6 months (10), age >70 years (5); physical: S_3 or jugular vein distension (11), aortic stenosis (3); ECG: non-sinus or premature atrial contraction (7), premature ventricular contractions >50 mmHg, K <3.0 mmol/l; General: pO_2 <60 mmHg, pCO_2 >50 mmHg, K <3.0 mmol/l, HCO_3 <20 mmol/l, blood urea nitrogen >50 mg/dl, Cr >3.0 mg/dl, hepatic (SGOT increase), bedridden (3); Operation: peritoneal, thoracic (3), aortic, emergency (4)

†Myocardial infarction: <6 months (10), >6 months (5); angina: class III (10), class IV (20); unstable angina: <6 months; pulmonary edema: (5), <1 week (10); valvular: critical aortic stenosis (20); arrythmia: non-sinus or premature ventricular contractions 5/min (5); general: poor medical (5), age >70 years (5), emergency (10)

Postoperative monitoring and specific interventions directed towards pain and anxiety are significant aspects of ICU care. Postoperative cardiac surgery patients who underwent standard anesthetic induction and analgesia maintenance in the operating room and management in the ICU with a precisely controlled analgesia regimen of sufentanil (5–10 µg/kg followed by 1µg/kg/h), compared to morphine (2 mg/kg), demonstrated a decreased incidence and severity of subsequent myocardial ischemia in Mangano and colleagues' evaluation of 106 patients[15].

Interventional analgesia techniques, such as the lumbar or thoracic epidural catheter, provide superior pain control without the adverse cardiopulmonary side-effects of systemically administered narcotics. This technique, used by Kirsch and associates[16] in patients with myasthenia gravis undergoing trans-sternal thymectomy, resulted in a decreased pain score (from 7.0 to 3.5), a decreased early (< 8 h) post-operative supplemental opioid-requirement regimen (from 0.22 to 0.12 mg/kg morphine equivalents) and improved pulmonary status, i.e. increased functional vital capacity (from 34 to 55%) and decreased respiratory rate. However, late (> 8 h) postoperative analgesia requirements and duration of intubation were not affected[16].

Anesthesia expertise allows precise intervention and control of anxiety using benzodiazepines, sedative-hypnotics, barbiturates, major tranquilizers or antidepressants for perioperative sedation. Similarly, analgesia is achieved using narcotics and local anesthesia administered by standard incremental dosing, continuous infusion, intravenous or intramuscular therapy, peripheral nerve blockade, epidural catheter, the transdermal route or patient-controlled routes.

RISK FACTORS

Predisposition to postoperative complications may be predicted by analysis of certain high-profile patient populations. The general surgery operative mortality rate for elective cases is low, but higher in those with pre-existing cardiac, pulmonary or hepatic disease, malignancy, advanced age or sepsis, as reported by Greenburg and colleagues[17]. Similarly, in the particular hospital surveyed, patient volume may also be important. Luft and co-workers[18] suggested that mortality rates with open-heart surgery, vascular surgery, transurethral prostate resection and coronary artery bypass grafting may be 25–41%

lower in more active facilities than in hospitals with a surgical-procedure volume of fewer than 200 operations per category. A less dramatic difference was seen with other interventions such as hip arthroplasty and cholecystectomy, which showed no correlation at all between volume and mortality[18]. In this study of approximately 850 000 patients in 1500 hospitals, the mean death rate for representative surgical cases was 0.06 (± 0.052), and ranged from 0.009 for vagotomy and/or pyloroplasty for duodenal ulcer disease to 0.186 for abdominal aortic aneurysm resection and graft[18]. Collected series of surgical complications suggest a case mortality rate of 0.2–17.4% for 21 common surgical procedures (Table 2)[18-21].

Advanced age is perhaps the most commonly encountered condition associated with anesthesia risk. In a study by Lauven and associates[22] of 3905 geriatric patients over 60 years of age, many were found to have an increased incidence of chronic medical conditions including myocardial dysfunction (55%), respiratory abnormalities (41%), hypertension (32%), dysrhythmia (31%) and diabetes (18%), compared to younger patients. Patients over 75 years had a higher anesthesia risk classification, the American Society of Anesthesiologists III–IV (58% vs. 43%), with more severe complications (53%), and manifested a similar elective, but increased emergency mortality rate (25 vs. 18%), compared to younger patients[22].

Specific disease conditions, medications or anatomical variables may be problematic in the postoperative period. For instance, myasthenia gravis often affects the recuperative ability of patients; however, the mortality rate with this disorder (4.8%) has improved as a result of perioperative assessment and intensive care post-thymectomy, based on Crucitti and colleagues' evaluation of 103 patients[23]. Hypertrophic cardiomyopathy patients may be adversely affected by the anesthesia agents isoflurane and halothane, resulting in ventricular tachycardia and sudden cardiac death, which may be prevented by a 24–48-h ICU monitoring period as suggested by Okuyama and associates[24]. Cystic fibrosis patients require comprehensive care related to bronchospasm, secretory plugging, pneumothorax, nutrition, hydration and infectious disease issues, as described by Cole and Cotton[25], which may be addressed with medications such as aerosolized aminoglycosides.

Pharmacological intervention such as long-term corticosteroid therapy may have an adverse impact on postoperative recovery. Steroids used for bronchopulmonary compared to non-pulmonary conditions

Table 2 Absolute mortality rates for 21 selected general surgical procedures: mortality rate is number of deaths per number of patients. Data from references 18–21

Procedure	Luft et al. (1979)	Flood et al. (1984)	Sloan et al. (1986)	Hannan et al. (1989)	Cumulative (1979–89)
Abdominal aortic aneurysm resection	0.1862	0.1550		0.1798	0.1739
Lower extremity amputation		0.1440			0.1440
Partial gastrectomy				0.1229	0.1229
Vascular surgery	0.1070				0.1070
Biliary tract surgery	0.0859				0.0859
Cardiac surgery	0.0810				0.0810
Colectomy	0.0687			0.0602	0.0681
Nephrectomy	0.0620				0.0620
Hip fixation		0.0800	0.0400		0.0788
Coronary artery bypass	0.0467		0.0430	0.0451	0.0458
Gastric ulcer surgery		0.0430			0.0430
Pelvis/femur fixation		0.0395			0.0395
Colon surgery		0.0320			0.0320
Vagotomy	0.0271				0.0271
Cholecystectomy, common bile duct incision	0.0264				0.0264
Morbid obesity surgery			0.0160		0.0160
Total hip arthroplasty	0.0159	0.015			0.0155
Cholecystectomy	0.0099	0.0110		0.0139	0.0104
Spinal fusion			0.0060		0.0060
Mastectomy			0.0030		0.0030
Hysterectomy			0.0020		0.0020
Number of hospitals	1498	1200	521	270	3219
Number of patients	842 622	550 000	200 000	48 139	1 440 761

result in a ten-fold increase in complications owing to the longer duration of therapy (24 months vs. 6 months), which is a more significant variable than dose (0.5 mg/kg vs. 1.2 mg/kg) of hydrocortisone equivalent, according to Reding and co-workers' evaluation of 55 steroid-dependent patients[26].

Perhaps the most pervasive physiological issue is obesity. The incidence of respiratory, cardiovascular or metabolic complications is increased in obesity owing to inadequate physiological reserve of multiple organ systems; however, conditions may be optimized by preoperative evaluation, intraoperative monitoring and postoperative intensive care, as described by Perilli and colleagues[27] in their analysis of 55 morbidly obese patients.

INTENSIVE CARE

The proportion of health-care resources devoted to intensive care intervention has increased significantly. The medical ICU patient population of 2693 patients evaluated by Thibault and associates[28] was responsible for 37% of total hospital charges and 58% of mortality, which occurred predominantly in the aged, chronically ill who received active medical intervention. The actual intensive care mortality rate reported was half of that occurring on the general medical ward[28]. Functional outcome is the most significant issue in intensive care survivors. Ninety-four per cent of 1345 former ICU patients evaluated by Mundt and co-workers[29] survived to 6 months after ICU discharge, with the young able to return to work with slight disability, and older patients able to benefit from family interaction.

The goals of intensive care include preoperative assessment and risk evaluation, review of the intraoperative course and diligent postoperative monitoring to prevent suboptimal perfusion and oxygenation, according to a review by Smith[30].

The elderly may particularly benefit from perioperative (1–3 day) monitoring to avoid cardiopulmonary complications, such as cardiac failure, atelectasis and pneumonia, citing the experience of Kockerling and Gall[31]. Geriatric patients constituted 19% of the ICU population most often admitted after emergency (51%) medical, non-traumatic illness (87%), with a resultant mortality of 6.3%, from Frede and Lanter's series of 877 patients[32]. Long-term outcome was acceptable, with half of the patients returning home and surviving at least 2 years after their illness[32].

Significant findings were seen in 13% of 100 elderly patients evaluated by Older and Smith[33] during the preoperative period, resulting in postponement of surgery in 7% and outright cancellation in another 6% of the patients studied. Cardiac dysfunction indicated by a cardiac index of $< 2.2 \text{ l/min/m}^2$ was found in 11% of patients, renal dysfunction (creatinine clearance < 50 ml/min) in 19%, hypertension (mean arterial pressure >120 mmHg) in 15% and pulmonary dysfunction (shunt of 15%) in 10% of those elderly patients evaluated during the preoperative and 3-day postoperative periods[33].

The presence of a critical-care specialist may similarly improve outcome according to the ICU population of 439 patients evaluated by Brown and Sullivan[34], as evidenced by decreased ICU mortality (from 28 to 13%) and hospital mortality (from 36 to 25%) in a moderately ill population matched for illness severity using an acute physiology and chronic health evaluation (APACHE) score of 18–19[35]. The survival rate improves further if the ICU practitioner is 'on site' 24 h per day, compared to 'on call from home' coverage, as demonstrated in Li and colleagues' group of 954 patients[36]. This observation appears to be associated with an increase in invasive monitoring, specifically pulmonary artery catheterization (from 2 to 22%) and arterial pressure monitoring (from 0 to 9%)[36].

Likewise, the institution of a dedicated critical-care service demonstrates improved outcome, as studied in 212 medical ICU patients by Reynolds and associates[37], with a decrease in mortality from 74 to 54%. This population was matched for significant injury severity (APACHE 28–29) with the control population, and received increased aggressive intravascular monitoring, namely arterial (from 24 to 73%) and pulmonary artery (from 48 to 64%) catheterization[37]. However, a comparison by Hainer and Lawler[38] in 523 medical and coronary care patients between family practitioners and internal medical physicians suggested no difference in mortality (36% vs. 38%), charges ($US 4318 vs. $US 5155) or number of consultations obtained (0.8 vs. 0.7). This specific ICU patient population, however, was only of minor illness severity (APACHE II), which may have contributed to the good outcome[38].

There are both advantages and disadvantages to teaching-hospital environments. Zimmerman and colleagues' comparison[39] of 8269 teaching-service and 7028 non-teaching-hospital ICU patients, in an initial evaluation of teaching hospitals, suggests equivalent lengths of ICU stay but a two-fold increase in physicians consulted in the university-based teaching centers, which was associated with increased costs, mostly related to a 10.5% increase in diagnostic testing. However, the patient population treated in the teaching centers was younger, was more severely ill and had a better risk-adjusted outcome than that in the non-teaching centers[39].

Intensive care management often includes invasive hemodynamic monitoring, in addition to a specialized cognitive process. Preoperative hemodynamic evaluation of 41 nonagenarian patients using a pulmonary artery catheter by Schrader and co-workers[40] in the ICU demonstrated a 92% 6-month survival rate, noting an additional 2% mortality improvement. This approach of early invasive monitoring in the elderly was used by Del Guercio and Cohn[41], and resulted in operative clearance in all 148 patients, noting normal oxygen transport function in 13%, physiological alteration in 63% and severe functional deficiency in 23% of patients. This strategy allowed for the early diagnosis of cardiopulmonary impairment and manipulation of cardiac parameters including preload, contractility and afterload, and thereby improved the patients' preoperative status.

Elderly patients often demonstrate some type of cardiopulmonary impairment indicated by a decreased cardiac index and increased pulmonary vascular resistance during the 'preoperative tune-up', as reported by Yamanaka and colleagues[42] in a group of 151 patients with esophageal cancer. This condition may be improved by the administration of vasopressors such as dopamine or inotropic agents such as dobutamine. A cardiopulmonary profile obtained through preoperative pulmonary artey catheterization may be a predictor of length of ICU stay and mortality. Del Guercio and co-workers[43] reported that a mortality rate of between 0 and 7.5% and length of ICU stay ranging from 1.5 to 27.7 days were associated with a pulmonary capillary wedge pressure of 6.3–12.2 mmHg, right-ventricular stroke work of 4.1–9.9 g, pulmonary vascular resistance of 169–319 (dyn × s × cm^{-5}), and an intrapulmonary shunt of 11–19% in a group of 100 high-risk elective cases. Preoperative 'fine tuning' occurred in half of these patients, who received volume expansion (37%), inotropic support (23%) or aggressive pulmonary care (17%)[43].

The use and effectiveness of aggressive ICU care for the elderly are often questioned. Margulies and associates[44] evaluated a group of 140 nonagenarians, compared to 5652 patients who were less than 90 years of age. The nonagenarians had both an increased simplified acute physiology score (SAPS) (11.1 vs. 8.6) and an increased hospital mortality rate (17.1% vs. 5.3%), while the ICU mortalities were similar[44]. The authors concluded that age alone was not a criterion to preclude ICU use, even though a mortality difference was noted. Chelluri and colleagues[45] evaluated outcome for those in the septagenarian age range with 54 patients of over 75 years, and 43 patients of 65–74 years. They found equivalent hospital lengths of stay, mortality rates and hospital charges[45]. Thus, critical care is best individualized to the specific condition.

QUALITY IMPROVEMENT

The issue of cost-effectiveness is often raised, but charges for preoperative ICU stay and monitoring are minimal, compared to those for the extensive hospital stays encountered after significant postoperative complications occur. This aggressive preoperative monitoring and interventional approach were used by Berlauk and colleagues[46], and included fluid-loading, inotropic support and afterload reduction, which were accompanied by decreased intraoperative events, postoperative morbidity and mortality (1.5% vs. 9.9%) but no decrease in hospital stay or costs.

There is an obvious need to quantify performance and effectiveness of care. Zimmerman and associates[47] evaluated 3672 ICU admissions for efficiency, measured as risk-adjusted survival and the ratio of actual to predicted length of stay. They concluded that superior facilities were not different in structural or organizational components, but had strong medical and nursing leadership, emphasizing co-operation[47].

Rapoport and colleagues devised a method for assessing the clinical performance of an ICU, i.e. the observed hospital mortality rate/predicted mortality rate, and the economic performance, i.e. the weighted hospital day index, recording length of stay equivalent to the actual main resource use compared to resource use predicted by regression analysis including severity of illness and percentage of surgical patients[48]. Interestingly, most hospitals studied were similar in performance with <1 standard deviation from the mean, suggesting that good clinical and economic performance is achievable in all health-care centers[48].

CARDIAC

A significant proportion of ICU resources is dedicated to addressing acute or chronic cardiac dysfunction. Preoperative evaluation that revealed left-ventricular dysfunction had direct implications for operative risk in the 183 coronary artery bypass graft patients studied by

Goenen and co-workers[49]. Abnormal left-ventricular function was found in 69% of patients evaluated. These patients had an increased incidence of myocardial infarction, inotropic requirements, intra-aortic balloon pump placement and arrythmia, and longer ICU stays[49]. Mortality, however, was equivalent to that in patients without left-ventricular dysfunction.

Postoperative concerns include new-onset arrythmia or ischemia. Postoperative atrial fibrillation often occurred in those predisposed by age (over 60 years), smoking as found in 79%, hypertension as found in 44% and malignancy, in Gibbs and colleagues' evaluation of 43 SICU patients[50]. This arrythmia usually began early in the postoperative phase (2.8 days), lasted on average 2.1 days and had no adverse effect on outcome[50].

Patients with a prior myocardial infarction had a 6% infarction risk in the postoperative period and were predisposed by a history of hypertension, perioperative hypotension or anesthesia time more than 3 h, according to Steen and associates' analysis of 587 patients[51]. The mortality rate was 4.2% overall with perioperative myocardial infarction, and reinfarction had a graded incidence of 27% if the operative intervention occurred less than 3 months from prior myocardial infarction, of 11% if 3–6 months, and of 5% if intervention was more than 6 months after previous myocardial infarction[51].

The incidence of intraoperative cardiac arrest in non-cardiothoracic patients was 0.015% or 24 of 162 661 cases reviewed by Girardi and Barie[52]. The post-resuscitation survival rate was 62% initially with nine (38%) patients surviving to hospital discharge. Predictors of mortality included the need for persistent vasopressor or inotropic support, or arrest duration of 15 min or greater[52].

The elderly (more than 70 years) are also at risk for complications after cardiac surgery, specifically coronary artery bypass grafting or valve replacement. The preoperative evaluation often reveals impaired pulmonary and renal function, requiring more aggressive mechanical ventilation and inotropic support during the postoperative course[53]. Mortality in the elderly population owing to more frequent neurological events, pneumonia and sepsis may be minimized by perioperative monitoring in the ICU[53].

Interventional care of the elderly with acute myocardial infarction was examined by McClellan and colleagues[54], who demonstrated a 5% increase in survival when comparing high-volume urban facilities with lower-volume rural facilities. However, when controlling for less access to interventional therapy including catheterization, angioplasty and revascularization, the actual mortality rate was only 0.6–1.0% better for high-volume facilities[54]. The slight improvement in outcome in high-volume facilities is related to early aggressive therapeutic intervention, and less so to early diagnostic procedures.

Assessment of preoperative anesthesia myocardial risk begins with non-invasive echocardiographic imaging[55]. Echocardiography performed in B mode (gray scale) or dynamic real time provides qualitative estimates of chamber size and thickness. Vascular integrity and function are assessed by Doppler (duplex) quantification of volume and direction of flow by either transesophageal or transthoracic routes.

Nuclear medical imaging allows estimation of current active ischemia or past myocardial infarction. These studies use flow-directed tracers ('hot' label) concentrated proportionally to blood flow. Technetium (^{99}Tc) studies label areas of past infarction by binding to calcium deposits in areas of infarction and necrosis. Thallium (^{201}Tl) is distributed to areas of active blood flow and delineates areas of ischemia in low-flow areas. The addition of a stress state using exercise, or administration of dipyramidole or dobutamine, allows for vasodilatation of coronary vasculature to evaluate the reversibility of ischemia.

Clinical validation of these cardiac testing strategies in the critically ill patient should be reviewed. Non-invasive determination of cardiac output was achieved by Kessler and Enders[56] using impedance cardiography, which correlated well ($r = 0.933$) with the thermodilution methodology in a group of ten post-cardiopulmonary bypass patients. This technique suggested that myocardial 'stunning' occurs after cardiac bypass, with a 26% decrease in cardiac output at 24 h, improving to a 6% decrease by 48 h[56]. This cardiac output measurement allows for close monitoring of fluid status and subsequent cardiac function.

Emergency echocardiography may also be used in the perioperative ICU patient. Ischemic dysfunction was revealed by echocardiogram in over half of the 297 cardiac surgery patients in Viossat and colleagues' study[57], while only 5% went on to have a normal cardiac catheterization. This population was managed medically in two-thirds and surgically in one-third of cases[57]. The addition of Doppler methodology improved sensitivity to 93% in the setting of cardiovascular dysfunction[58]. Echocardiography was associated with a minimal false-positive rate (1.9%), comparable to cardiac catheterization, for the diagnosis of valvular insufficiency, with similar mortality rates for underlying conditions (3.6% vs. 3.3%) in Carreras and associates' study of 306 patients[58].

Nuclear cardiology imaging provides both preoperative assessment of risk and perioperative diagnosis of myocardial infarction. Screening tests performed in Eagle and co-workers' study[59] of a high-prevalence population were predictive of outcome, with a positive test associated with a 37% complication rate and a negative test with no complications in that group of 111 cardiac disease patients. Reversibility of the cardiac uptake was also associated (44%) with postoperative cardiac complications, whereas a fixed defect without reperfusion was not associated (0%) with these complications[59]. Perioperative myocardial events have been documented by technetium ^{99}Tc labeling in cardiac bypass grafting patients, with new infarction in 5% of patients and reversible ischemia in 16%, in the ICU setting in Raff and colleagues' group of 18 perioperative patients[60]. Patients with permanent cardiac pacemakers often warrant ICU monitoring. Surgical intervention may result in pacemaker malfunction secondary to loss of pacing threshold as a result of drugs of hypokalemia, ventricular fibrillation owing to electrode conduction abnormalities, or to spontaneous reprogramming owing to electrocautery[61]. Likewise, certain cardiac conduction abnormalities such as atrioventricular block may benefit from prophylactic transvenous pacemaking placement in the ICU[62,63].

Valve replacement surgery for endocarditis warrants aggressive postoperative care. Arena and co-workers[64] reported on a 25-patient group who had aortic valve replacement (73%) or mitral valve replacement (27%), associated with a 4% hospital mortality rate, an 8% 1-year mortality rate and an 87% actuarial 5-year survival.

Novel approaches to cardiothoracic ICU care emphasize care of high-risk coronary artery bypass graft patients. Eleftariades and colleagues[65] evaluated 83 patients with advanced ischemic cardiomyopathy having a mean left-ventricular ejection fraction of 25% (range 10–30%), who presented with congestive heart failure (52%), angina (49%) and arrythmia (30%). The high-risk groups had increased mortality in 8.4% (7 of 83) of patients, while standard patients had a 3.3% (2 of 61) mortality rate; in this study, the internal mammary artery to left-anterior descending artery bypass graft was the most common (82%) procedure chosen[65]. This analysis suggested that high-risk coronary artery bypass graft surgery can be safely performed with 87% 1-year actual survival associated with a significant improvement in left-ventricular ejection fraction (from 25 to 33%) and functional classification[65].

Comparisons of survival should emphasize a risk-adjusted approach to analysis. Hattler and associates[66] examined outcome in patients who underwent preoperative risk stratification using the Society of Thoracic Surgeons' database ranging from low (0–5%), through 5–10%, 10–20% and 20–30%, to high-risk (>30%) groups. This risk stratification correlated with morbidity and length of stay, with the high-risk (>30%) group suffering the most complications (28%), including ventilator dependence (33%), renal failure and cardiac arrest (17%), while the moderate-risk (>20%) group demonstrated 24.3% mortality[66].

Overall mortality in the cardiothoracic surgery population was 19.6%, as reported from Kollef and co-workers' evaluation of 472 patients[67] and prolonged ventilator dependence occurred in 22.7% (107 of 472) of cases. Correlates of mortality were an organ system failure index of >3, associated by univariate analysis to the presence of anti-biotic resistant infection, aortic cross clamp time >1.25 h, ventilator associated pneumonia and APACHE II score >30[67].

The intra-aortic balloon pump is used as mechanical support in cardiac failure until medical recovery occurs or surgical therapy is instituted. The critically ill patient (Goldman class III–IV, Detsky class III) with a complication rate of 14–56% and mortality rate of 21–76% has been shown to benefit most from aggressive intervention, such as the prophylactic use of the intra-aortic balloon pump in high-risk patients[10,12,68]. Georgeson and colleagues' group of ten critically ill patients[68], however, was already predisposed to poor outcome, accord-ing to their baseline medical condition and significant complications, predominantly vascular in nature (18%), which resulted in surgical inter-vention in half of the patients and amputation of an extremity in 6%.

The ventricular-assist device is used in patients with myocardial failure refractory to the intra-aortic balloon pump and vasopressors. Adamson and associates[69] recommended its use in patients who failed to wean from cardiac bypass (65%), or required ICU care (28%) or cardiac transplant (7%). Although the ventricular-assist device is associated with high mortality (72%), in this sample of 43 patients, approximately one-half of those discharged had a normal recovery[69]. Correlation with good recovery included early use, biventricular sup-port, transplantation and operator expertise[69].

Commonly used ventricular-assist devices including the Novocor® (Baxter, division of Novocor Oakland, CA, USA) left-ventricular-assist system and the Thoratec® (Thoratec Lab Corporation, Berkley, CA, USA) ventricular-assist device are predominantly utilized as a 'bridge to transplant'. Patients that survive the initial ICU course often do well in the long term, according to an 18-patient study reported by Mulcahy and colleagues[70]. There was 94% (17 of 18) 5-year survival with 59% (10 of 17) returning to full-time employment and 65% (11 of 17) living with no restriction of daily activity[70].

PULMONARY

High-risk pulmonary patients often benefit from ICU care featuring preoperative medical regimen optimization, operative fluid titration, minimization of nitrous oxide-induced atelectasis, pain management or pulmonary toilet for 48–96 h postoperatively, according to Slinger[71].

High-risk patients include the elderly, and those with myasthenia gravis or chronic obstructive pulmonary disease or undergoing pulmonary resection. The geriatric (over 70 years) thoracotomy patient has a 7.5% mortality and a 17% complication rate and, in select cases, benign-disease survival is 100% with careful ICU management, as suggested by Ebner and co-workers' analysis of 53 cases[72]. Patients with myasthenia gravis could be extubated within 12 h of thymectomy, in spite of a 50% reduction in vital capacity in 100% of the patients maintained in a closely monitored ICU setting in Gorback and colleagues' series of 14 patients[73].

Chronic obstructive pulmonary disease patients undergoing resection for stage Ia lung cancer have a decreased 5-year survival rate (from 53 to 35%), compared to normal patients, with advanced age and the presence of cardiopulmonary dysfunction worsening prognosis[74]. A carefully staged approach to anesthesia and postoperative care, based on pulmonary functional capacity and the presence of hypoxemia or hypercarbia, resulted in 0% mortality in Milledge and Nunn's 12-patient sample[75]. Patients with minor lung disease with decreased vital capacity and normal arterial blood gas results benefited from chest physiotherapy and prophylactic antibiotics; however, those with significant lung disease with decreased vital capacity and hypoxemia required supplemental oxygen therapy, and those with severe disease with hypercarbia in addition often required mechanical ventilation postoperatively[75].

Thoracic surgical intervention is often preceded by pulmonary function testing to predict the success of lung resection therapy. The forced expiratory volume for 1 s (FEV_1) is the reference standard, with 0.8–1.0 l the suggested minimum to wean successfully post-lobectomy, whereas a volume between 1.0 and 2.0 l often requires further investigation to decide the proper surgical option[74,76]. Auxiliary studies such as a differential perfusion lung scan or exercise testing may suggest a more conservative surgical approach, such as wedge resection or segmentectomy, as opposed to lobectomy or pneumonectomy for pulmonary malignancy[76].

The predictive nature of preoperative pulmonary function testing has recently been challenged by Kearnery and colleagues[77]. Standards such as hypercarbia, desaturation or FEV_1 less than 1 l have not proved predictive; however, age greater than 60 years, male sex, tobacco abuse, pneumonectomy or a decrease in postoperative FEV_1 by 0.2 l have correlated with adverse outcome[77].

The postoperative risk of thoracotomy is well described. Thoracotomy for malignancy was associated with a 39% pulmonary complication rate of which two-thirds were major and one-third were minor, resulting in a 6% mortality rate as reported in Busch and associates' series[78] of 104 patients. The likelihood of pulmonary complications increases with chemotherapy or poor nutritional status, which are also associated with subsequent cardiac dysfunction[78].

Cardiac disturbance after thoracotomy is common, and may be predicted by preoperative variables. In a study by von Knorring and colleagues[79] the presence of postoperative tachyarrhythmia, atrial tachycardia, fibrillation or flutter was noted in 87% of 94 patients, and was accompanied by ischemia in 4% and myocardial infarction in 1%. Mortality increased eight-fold to 17% if the arrhythmia was recurrent[79]. Predisposition to cardiac events may be strongly predicted ($p < 0.001$) by a positive exercise stress test or operative hypotension, and more weakly predicted by prior cardiomegaly, pneumonectomy or electrocardiographic changes[79]. Early diagnosis and therapy of postoperative arrhythmia may be beneficial.

Outcome from long-term (more than 29-day) mechanical ventilation was reported by Gracey and co-workers[80] in a study of 104 postsurgical patients. The average length of stay was 21.5 ± 14.2 days prior to tracheostomy. Overall ICU survival was 51.7%, with 67% of patients remaining alive at 1 year and 56% at 3 years[80]. Therefore, even in this severely ill group, mortality tends to plateau between 1 and 3 years after discharge.

RENAL

Renal failure encountered during an ICU stay often precludes significant recovery. The presence of an abnormal preoperative creatinine level, concurrent valve surgery or coronary artery surgery, or advanced age predicted 77% of acute renal failure cases in 57% of cardiac surgery patients studied by Corwin and associates[81]. The resulting renal failure was associated with significant increases in hospital length of stay, morbidity and mortality[81].

Acute hemodialysis in a group of 21 elderly (over 72 years) SICU patients was associated with a mortality rate of 86% in Mukau and Latimer's study[82]. Preoperative evaluation suggested that patients with an abnormal creatinine clearance (< 41 ml/min) had a mortality rate of 100%, compared to 80% in those with a more normal creatinine clearance. Predisposition to renal failure was determined by the presence of sepsis or multisystem organ failure (100%), a hypotension episode (43%), or administration of nephrotoxic drugs or dye (33%)[82]. Acute renal failure in this ICU population usually presented as fluid overload (95%), and responded well to early dialysis[82].

Acute renal failure was evaluated in 242 elderly patients by Druml and colleagues[83], noting risk factors for subsequent dialysis of a creatinine level of >6 mg/dl, anuria, a blood urea nitrogen level of >120 mg/dl, ventilator dependence or septicemia. The mortality rate was significant at 61%, but a decrease in mortality from 70 to 50% was noted with improvements in care from 1970 to 1994, even with an increase in disease severity[83].

Early detection of ICU renal dysfunction may be achieved by the use of renal duplex ultrasound scanning, measuring the renal resistive index or the ratio of the difference between systolic and diastolic pressure over diastolic pressure[84]. This measure of renal perfusion, if decreased, correlated with renal dysfunction, hemodialysis, length of

ICU and hospital stay and mortality in Platt and colleagues' evaluation[84] of 42 liver transplant patients.

The renal transplant population is often considered for ICU care and intervention. Sadaghdar and co-workers[85] evaluated 72 renal transplant patients admitted for postoperative complications in two-thirds of cases associated with a 16% mortality rate, while those admitted for routine postoperative care in one-third of cases had a mortality rate of 4%. This population had a hospital mortality rate of 14%, a two-fold increase compared to the general surgery population[85].

IMMUNOLOGY

Wound healing is a significant part of the postoperative recovery phase. Wound complications were found by Norris and colleagues[86] to increase hospital length of stay, morbidity and mortality. Patients were predisposed to wound infection by age, diabetes, malnutrition, obesity or chronic illness, and the infection improved if given adequate perfusion and oxygen delivery[86].

Wound infection was found in 16% of 1451 colorectal oncological surgery patients predisposed by anemia and hypothermia, as reported by Fass[87]. This condition is often reversible with aggressive ICU care and appropriate systemic antibiotics and surgical debridement, yet may result in a 10–25% mortality rate[87].

In a study of 221 consecutive adult cardiac surgical patients evaluated by Ulicny and associates[88], correlates to sternotomy infection included age, weight, preoperative ICU requirement, repeat sternotomy, internal mammary artery graft, postoperative bleeding and cardiac arrest. Sternal wound infections occurred in 2.7% of patients, and were predicted by abnormal preoperative nutritional indices (decreased prealbumin, transferrin, retinol binding protein), as well as increased acute-phase reactants (C-reactive protein, α_1-acid glycoprotein) or a delayed hypersensitivity panel[88].

INFECTIOUS DISEASE

The control of infectious complications in the ICU begins with acknowledging the health-care provider as the most likely vector of transmission from the patient reservoir. The single most effective maneuver to decrease infection is handwashing with an antimicrobial soap. A paradoxical increase in organisms has been noted with hand-washes of less than 10 s[89]. Maki[89] noted that, in a comparison of 10% povidone–iodine and 4% chlorhexidine, with non-medicated soap as the control, the antimicrobial compounds were associated with a 50% decline in nosocomial infection.

Postoperative pulmonary infection can often be predicted by preoperative culture assessment in those predisposed by a history of smoking or abnormal pulmonary function testing[90]. In a study by Carrel and colleagues[90], 31% of 100 patients with a positive sputum culture for a pathogenic species developed pneumonia, compared to 1% of those with negative sputum cultures. The incidence of nosocomial pneumonia was 16% in a SICU population of 582 intubated patients studied by Konrad and associates[91]. Postoperative pneumonia was associated with mechanical ventilation for 3 days or more, altered level of consciousness, vasopressor use, barbiturate use, antiarrhythmic therapy, pulmonary disease and, less commonly, male sex, American Society of Anesthesiologists (ASA) grade IV assessment and smoking history[91].

Surgical wound infection may be predicted by examination of a risk-factor scale devised by Culver and co-workers[92], consisting of: 1, ASA grade III, IV, V assessment; 2, contaminated operation; or 3, prolonged surgery. The incidence of infection was 1.5% for those free of risk factors, 3% for those with a risk index of 1, 7% for a risk index of 2 and 13% if all risk factors were present[92]. Intra-abdominal sepsis is a particularly severe infectious syndrome found in the critically ill patient. This syndrome presented with an abnormal abdominal examination, bacteremia or sepsis syndrome, and was confirmed through ultrasound or computed tomography, with an associated sensitivity of 80–95% in Sinanan and colleagues' study[93] of 71 patients. Early directed operative abdominal exploration revealed an infection or ischemic source in 81% of patients studied, and a decreased mortality rate from 90 to 51%[93].

Recently, gastrointestinal tract decontamination using a combination of non-absorbable antibiotics and antifungal agents has been suggested to decrease intra-abdominal and pulmonary infections in the critically ill patient. Hartenauer and associates' prospective cross-over design trial of 200 patients[94] suggested a decrease in Gram-negative rod colonization, pneumonia and urinary tract infection, but mortality was not improved. Similarly, in Gastinne and co-workers' multicenter trial[95] of 445 ventilated patients, bacterial colonization was decreased but without a reduction in pneumonia cases or mortality. The issue of gut decontamination and its effect on outcome warrants further study.

Studies of human monoclonal immunoglobulin-M antibodies such as HA-1A have had mixed results. The French National Committee for the Evaluation of Centoxin[96] studied 600 patients, with 75% manifesting an identified site of Gram-negative infection and 39% progressing to bacteremia. Mortality was significant, ranging from 49% at 2 weeks into the hospital course to 61% by hospital discharge[96]. Interestingly, the relative risk of mortality was increased by 1.32 for those with non-Gram-negative bacteria in the treatment group. Early sepsis was recently evaluated by Le Gall and colleagues[97], from a 1458-patient database, occurring at an incidence of 9.8% associated with a two-fold increase in mortality (from 19.6 to 48.0%).

GASTROINTESTINAL

A diverse group of gastrointestinal disturbances may benefit from ICU intervention. Acute biliary pancreatitis is a reversible condition caused by cholelithiasis, which often results in hemorrhagic necrosis. Early diagnosis with computed tomography, medical therapy with somatostatin and intervention directed at gallstone removal decreased the mortality rate (to 10%) in Gravero and co-workers' analysis[98] of acute biliary pancreatitis. A palliative or curative resection may be attempted to treat pancreatic malignancy, when localized to the periampullary region, according to Obertop and colleagues' experience with 75 patients[99]. The prognosis was adverse when vascular invasion was noted, or jaundice absent, resulting in a mortality rate of 8%. There was an initial mortality of 13% with exploratory laparotomy accompanied by pancreatoduodenectomy, after which survival was 94%; however, with total pancreatectomy, initial mortality was 0% and survival was 57%, suggesting that aggressive resection may be helpful[99].

Acute acalculous cholecystitis was caused by ischemia, resulting in gall bladder distention and necrosis found in patients predisposed by a prolonged ICU course, narcotic analgesics and total parenteral nutrition use, according to an analysis by Cornwell and associates[100]. Diagnosis was made by ultrasound, which revealed increased wall thickness (>4 mm), subserosal edema, sloughed mucosa, intramucosal gas and pericholecystic fluid. Therapeutic intervention includes percutaneous drainage and systemic broad-spectrum antibiotics in the critically ill ICU patient. Acalculous cholecystitis appears to be a disuse phenomenon of the gall bladder; therefore, early enteral feeding and avoidance of analgesics such as morphine sulfate with effects on the sphincter of Oddi may be beneficial.

Intestinal obstruction may result in significant hypovolemia and shock. Small intestinal conditions were caused by multiple serosal carcinomatosis lesions, with surgical palliation in 63% of patients, whereas colonic obstruction was caused by a single lesion, with palliation achieved in 100% of Aabo and colleagues' 41-patient series[101]. The diagnosis of intestinal obstruction was arrived at by a combination of clinical judgement, the occurrence of leukocytosis and the presence of fever, in Sarr and co-workers' series of 51 patients[102]. In this study of small bowel obstruction, preoperative diagnostic parameters only provided a sensitivity of 48% for complete, irreversible obstruction, whereas incomplete reversible conditions were more readily diagnosed, with 69% sensitivity[102]. Definitive diagnosis and therapy usually include laparotomy.

Extensive small intestine resection is more often required in males, by a 2 : 1 margin compared to females, and they are predisposed by superior mesenteric artery thrombus, tumor or invagination, according to Harju and Pessi's series of 43 patients[103]. Mortality is often cited to be 60%, but survival has been shown to improve in younger patients (under 60 years) and those with better nutrition (protein >8.0 mg/dl), an adequate leukocyte response (white blood cell count >20 000 cells/ml) and decreased blood loss (< 3.0 l)[103]. Surgery is required more often for small intestine (73%) than for colonic (27%) obstruction, based on Waclawiczek's group of 351 patients[104]. The rates of complications, including dehiscence, enterotomies, incisional hernia and ileus, were equivalent (26%), and ICU care reduced mortality by half (to 5%) for both conditions[104].

Massive gastrointestinal hemorrhage is often caused by diverticulitis in the young or angiodysplasia in the elderly population. An equal proportion of patients underwent medical or surgical management for lower gastrointestinal hemorrhage, and selective angiography assisted in two-thirds of 64 cases identified by Udien and colleagues[105]. Patients who were unable to tolerate selective mesenteric angiography had an 80% mortality rate, whereas those with positive angiographic results had a 14% mortality rate, and mortality was 0% in those with a negative angiographic evaluation[105].

Perhaps the single most ominous perioperative risk factor is the presence of advanced cirrhosis. In Garrison and associates' study[106], 100 cirrhotic patients who underwent non-shunt abdominal exploration had a complication rate of 30% and a mortality rate of 30%, with a range from 29% for biliary surgery to 55% for colectomy. Predictors of operative survival included blood loss, pulmonary failure, gastrointestinal bleeding and bacterial infection[106]. Portal hypertension shunt surgery is more common in the setting of gastrointestinal hemorrhage, ascites, renal failure, peritonitis, hepatolysis, cardiac failure and reoperation[107]. Mortality increases with age (over 50 years), hepatic fibrosis, hepatopathy, emergency intervention or a radiological shunt, according to Herrera Carranza and co-workers' evaluation of 26 patients[107].

A postoperative course of hepatic resection for pulmonary malignancy in cirrhotic patients resulted in hepatic failure in 19% of cases[91]. Preoperative liver function tests were not predictive of outcome, but lobectomy and extensive blood loss (>4 l) were associated with a fourfold (88%) increase in complications in Takenaka and colleagues' group of 126 patients[108]. Postoperative ICU care is paramount in the management of extensive hepatic resection, to avoid the lethal outcome of hepatic failure. In Cole and Ferguson's study[109], hepatic resection for metastatic colorectal carcinoma in 43 patients had a 23% morbidity rate, which was predicted by the extent of resection, length of operation and amount of blood transfused. In this study, however, all patients survived the surgery after a 3-day ICU stay[109].

Finally, the complication rate and length of hospital stay with penetrating or blunt hepatic trauma have been shown to decrease with ICU care, compared to ward management, owing to closer surveillance and defined management objectives, as demonstrated in Foco and colleagues' evaluation[110].

The pressure of asymptomatic peptic ulcer disease cannot be predicted by risk factors in the ICU patient, according to Rypins and associates' study of 72 patients[111]. Endoscopy before major surgery revealed ulceration in 14% and gastroduodenitis in 10% of patients, suggesting an augmented role of routine endoscopy and stress ulcer prophylaxis[111]. The pathogenesis of ICU stress ulcer is primarily a result of cellular ischemia with a secondary contribution of luminal acid. Studies such as that of Cook and colleagues[112], comparing single or combination therapy with routinely used stress ulcer agents such as H_2 antagonists, antacids, sucralfate, cytoprotective agents or parietal cell inhibitors, have failed to demonstrate a decrease in mortality.

ENDOCRINE

The presence of diabetes, with its adverse effects on cardiopulmonary reserve, renal function, wound healing and ability to resist infection, may complicate even routine surgery. Complications may be minimized by preoperative assessment, adequate insulin and glucose, and careful postoperative glucose monitoring, as suggested in Byyny's review[113].

Thyroid disease can also be problematic during postoperative management. Cardiopulmonary failure may be associated with thyroid malignancy, which had a 28% early and 49% late mortality rate postoperatively, as cited in Romanchishen's series of 47 advanced cases[114]. Early airway compromise owing to bleeding or swelling if surgical intervention is undertaken may be avoided through aggressive ICU monitoring. Hyperthyroidism is thought to be associated with atrial fibrillation; however, Siebers and colleagues' study of geriatric patients presenting with new-onset atrial fibrillation failed to demonstrate a single occult case of hyperthyroidism[115]. Hypothyroidism and its association with ventilation dependency have also been explored. Pandya and co-workers[116] suggest the incidence of hypothyroidism (decreased thyroxine, increased thyroid stimulating hormone) to be only 3%; this condition is more commonly found in the elderly, but seldom causes failure to wean, as a single variable usually cited in small case series.

Adrenal insufficiency is found in ICU patients predisposed by hypotension, sepsis, surgery or heparinization, as described by Dahlberg and associates[117] in a small series of 17 patients. Acute adrenal crisis presents with hemodynamic and temperature instability accompanied by a decrease in serum sodium and an increase in potassium[118]. Initial diagnosis is achieved by measurement of serum cortisol level, which is abnormal if less than 10–20 μg/dl, depending on the baseline state. The adrenocorticotropic hormone stimulation test, in which 0.25 mg of synthetic corticotropin is administered, requires a two-fold increase from baseline level denoting adequate response for confirmation.

NEUROLOGY

The presence of perioperative stroke is a catastrophic complication of surgery. This condition is associated with severe disability in elderly patients predisposed by cardiovascular disease, or suffering from vasospasm or embolic events. Monitoring in the ICU and therapy to prevent iatrogenic hypotension minimize postoperative cerebral vascular accidents, as suggested in Wong's review[119]. The mechanisms of postoperative cerebral damage found in cardiopulmonary bypass patients, according to Mravinac[120], include reperfusion, hyperemia and microemboli, resulting in a continuum of injury that spans from transient confusion to intracerebral hemorrhage. Monitoring of perioperative neural change by evoked potential or electroencephalography during neurosurgical procedures may predict and avert ischemic complications, according to Nau and colleagues[121].

Patients with chronic neuromuscular conditions are especially at risk for poor outcome. Cellerin and co-workers[122] classified 49 patients into those with progressive neuromuscular disease such as amyotrophic lateral sclerosis or multiple sclerosis associated with 85% 2-year mortality; primary muscle disorders or myopathies (55%); and non-progressive neuromuscular disease with 29% mortality. The overall mortality rate for the entire group was significant (60.3%), with over half requiring prolonged mechanical ventilation[122].

HEMATOLOGY

Conservative transfusion practices are warranted in view of the risk of viral disease. The risk was calculated as 1 : 100 for hepatitis C, 1 : 200–300 for hepatitis B and 1 : 40 000–1 000 000 for human immuno-deficiency virus, prior to 1988[123]. These risk estimates have been reduced somewhat, owing to better blood bank screening procedures. Strategies to minimize transfusion requirements include autologous transfusion from perioperative salvage; homologous transfusion from family members; the use of blood substitutes such as perfluorocarbons or modified hemoglobin; and pharmacological maneuvers to decrease loss, such as the use of desmopressin, or to stimulate production, such as the use of erythropoietin[124].

The benefits of blood transfusion, such as improvement in oxygen delivery, should be considered. The rate of postoperative complications and morbidity in a 2582 patient cardioplegia cohort was increased nearly 30% in the 97 patients who received crystalloid, whereas the 407 patients who received blood cardioplegia had fewer complications along with decreased hospital length of stay and wound infection incidence, according to Loop and colleagues' evaluation[125]. Lorentz and co-workers' clinical trial[126] of transfusion practices in 64 elective hip arthroplasty patients makes recommendations based on more than 500 ml of blood loss in 66% of the control patients. The best clinical strategy was preoperative autologous donation, which was attempted in 12% of patients with no transfusion risk; preoperative hemodilution, used in 9%, required 500 ml of transfusion, compared to perioperative autotransfusion used in 50%, which required half the blood transfusion volume[126]. Obviously, these strategies are less helpful in critically ill patients requiring emergency surgery.

NUTRITION

There has been significant debate regarding the role of nutrition in the ICU patient. Perioperative hyperalimentation has not been shown to improve mortality or to minimize complications in those with normal nutritional status, by the Veterans' Affairs Total Parenteral Nutrition Cooperative Study Group[127]. A subgroup of those 395 malnourished patients with moderate and severe malnutrition preoperatively, however, was shown to benefit from total parenteral nutrition[127]. In Detsky and colleagues' meta-analysis[128] of perioperative hyperalimentation delivered in 18 controlled clinical trials, a decrease in complications and mortality with sepsis isolated as a significant factor was found.

Assessment of nutritional status has progressed from delayed-type hypersensitivity skin testing, resulting in a 28% anergy rate in Brown and associates' study of 244 major surgery patients[129], arm-muscle circumference, and serum protein or albumin measurement with little correlation to outcome. The usefulness of more specific assessment techniques, such as measuring essential proteins like retinol-binding protein, instead of albumin, or metabolic rate measurement of carbon dioxide production to calculate respiratory quotient, remains to be established.

PSYCHIATRY

Postoperative delirium is a common phenomenon, found in 42% of patients in Dieckelmann and colleagues' study of 92 patients[130], and usually occurs between 2 and 7 days after surgery. A predictive model based on age, ventilatory status and arterial oxygen tension was used with 78% accuracy to predict the incidence of delirium[130]. Etiology of delirium may be related to disturbance in circadian periodicity, or to increased β-endorphin and cortisol owing to exogenous opiate interactions with the hypothalamic–pituitary axis, as postulated by McIntosh and co-workers[131]. Postoperative alterations in mental status are most commonly classified as delirium, followed by perceptual changes or confusion.

Factors associated with postoperative confusion from Sveinsson's study[132] of 22 patients include sleep deprivation found in 93% of patients with the condition, age, disease severity and antecedent psychiatric illness. The first factor may be exacerbated by ICU care; therefore, early discharge to a more controlled setting may be desirable. Savageau and associates[133] evaluated neuropsychiatric dysfunction associated with cardiac surgery, as measured by the Wechsler Adult Intelligence Scale, and demonstrated an 11–17% decrease in cognitive function.

Preoperative considerations associated with delirium include age more than 60 years, end-diastolic pressure more than 30 mmHg, cardiomegaly and hypertension; perioperative issues include prolonged operative time (>7 h) and cross-clamp time (>2 h), excess blood loss (>2 l), difficult intubation and inotropic-agent or balloon-pump use; and postoperative findings include electrolyte abnormalities and prolonged ICU course, resulting in significant depression and abnormal behavior[133].

SURGICAL SUBSPECIALTY

Plastic surgery patients often require ICU care to maintain the flap viability. Free-flap surgical procedures commonly involve the lower extremities (57%) or the head–neck (25%) region, and the types of flap commonly employed are the latissimus dorsi (40%) and Chinese (28%) variations, based on Legre and colleagues' experience with 106 general patients[134]. The success rate for all free flaps was 87% in this study, and it was suggested that a large proportion of failures may be avoided by close ICU monitoring of flap viability[134].

Urology patients often require ICU care after extensive oncological surgery. Mortality with radical cystectomy was reduced from 20 to 3%, based on an intensive care regimen consisting of adequate bowel preparation, cardiac medication management including anticoagulation, digitalis, systemic antibiotics and hyperalimentation, and deep venous thrombosis prophylaxis according to Ackermann and Ebert[135]. These findings were confirmed in Hendry's study[136], which suggested a reduction in mortality from 11% in the 1970s to 2%, based on improved ICU care and surgical techniques.

Vascular surgery patients, almost by definition, have diffuse vessel disease along with other organ system dysfunction. Cardiac risk in the setting of peripheral vascular disease is significant, with 16% of patients suffering a lethal myocardial infarction according to Jivegard and co-workers' evaluation of 117 postoperative patients[137]. The range may extend from 3 to 75%, based on a combination of factors including systemic hypotension (mean arterial pressure <90 mmHg), cardiac failure, thigh ischemia, hemoglobin level more than 14 g/dl or prior myocardial infarction within 4 weeks, according to Kepiantalo and associates' study of 40 amputees[138]. Non-invasive Doppler monitoring of segmental blood pressure may be predictive of amputation success. Healing was associated with proximal thigh pressure of 100 mmHg and distal calf pressure of 68 mmHg, whereas failure to heal was noted at levels of 60 mmHg and 35 mmHg, respectively, with a 40% reduction in blood flow[138].

Abdominal aortic aneurysm surgery often has a catastrophic outcome in emergency cases, and poses a notable risk in elective cases. Abdominal aortic aneurysm reported by Kortmann and Becker[139] in the geriatric patient was associated with a greater mortality risk: asymptomatic 0%, symptomatic 25%, and 46% with rupture in this 97-case sample. Patients are at risk with concurrent coronary artery disease, and techniques such as early ultrasound diagnosis and ICU care have been shown to reduce mortality from 44 to 16%[139].

Thoracoabdominal aortic aneurysm care was studied in 88 patients by Schepens and colleagues[140], identifying a cumulative mortality of 11.4% if aortic cross-clamping occurred. A logistic regression model using the factors age and preoperative creatinine level was able to predict the need for postoperative dialysis, while a Cox proportional hazard model showed the need for dialysis to be a risk factor for late death[140] after the ICU stay.

During intensive care of the patient with an abdominal aortic aneurysm, 80% developed a single complication while 59% developed multiple complications, resulting in a mortality rate of 7% in Campbell and co-workers' 45-patient series[141]. These complications were unpredictable, delaying recovery in elective cases, and included oliguria (69%), hypertension (44%), hypotension (38%), pulmonary dysfunction (27%) and hypoxia (22%)[141]. In another study, the complication rate with an aneurysm reconstruction was minimal: ICU care of 3 days or more was required in only 14% of patients in Bjerkelund and colleagues' series of 109 patients[142]. A mortality rate of 6%, however, remained even in carefully selected cases[142].

Burn patients require intensive care intervention based on the extent of the burn or the presence of inhalation injury. Inhalation injury occurred in 26% (330 of 1256) of patients analyzed by Rue and co-workers[143], and was associated with a greater extent of burn (51% vs. 18%) and a six-fold increase in mortality (29% vs. 5%). Development of advanced care methods was responsible for a decrease in mortality from 41.4% in 1980–84 to 29.4% in 1985–90[143].

PHYSICAL THERAPY

Physical therapy and rehabilitation are often neglected during the ICU course. Physical therapy addresses pulmonary care through early mobilization, positioning, percussion and vibration, and neuromuscular care through early ambulation, encouraging active and passive range of motion, and splinting extremities to prevent diverse atrophy, according to Dean and Ross's review[144].

Perhaps the most significant issue is the prevention of pressure sores, which occurred in 5% of those hospitalized in Allman and colleagues' series of 634 patients[145]. This risk profile was increased almost three-fold (to 12%) in those with risk factors including fecal incontinence, diarrhea, fracture, bladder catheterization, decreased weight, dementia and hypoalbuminemia[145].

The use of specialty beds may decrease the incidence of skin breakdown in selected patients. The use of an air-fluidized bed protocol by Allman and associates[146] resulted in a 5.6-fold decrease in breakdown surface area for both small (less than 1.2 cm²: 45 to 75% improvement) and large (1.2–5.3 cm²: 29 to 62% improvement) decubiti in 62 patients.

Fink and co-workers[147] suggested that the use of an oscillating bed may reduce the incidence of tracheobronchitis and pneumonia, as well as the days of ventilation, ICU stay and hospital stay, based on their group of 106 patients.

Deep venous thrombosis (DVT) is associated with significant morbidity and mortality. Diagnosis has evolved from impedance plethysmography and fibrinogen I scanning[125] to duplex ultrasound with Doppler capability and contrast venography, while therapy examines new low-molecular-weight heparin regimens and defines the role of intravenous filters.

The standard DVT prophylaxis is twice-daily heparin doses of 5000 u administered by a subcutaneous route, which resulted in a significant decrease (from 34 to 6%) in subsequent lower-extremity thrombosis, but with equivalent bleeding complication rates, in Cerrato and colleagues' study of 110 elective neurosurgical patients[148]. DVT is the most common cause of morbidity and mortality in elective surgery and should be addressed in a protocolized fashion. The risk of complications of therapy in the setting of bleeding diathesis, underlying disease or new surgical anastomosis should be balanced against a catastrophic error of omission[149]. In Russell's protocol[149], high-risk patients were given warfarin and intravenous filters; moderate-risk patients were given heparin, dextran or pneumatic compression devices; and low-risk patients were treated with aspirin, support stockings and extremity elevation.

In Oster and associates' meta-analysis of various treatment strategies[150], a control regimen without prophylaxis yielded a 26.9% DVT rate, while support stockings, intermittent pneumatic compression and low-dose heparin yielded rates of 12.9%, 9.7% and 9%, respectively for subsequent DVT. The absolute rate of pulmonary embolism per 10 000 patients treated was 42 for no prophylaxis, 27 for intermittent pneumatic compression, 17 with elastic stockings, 15 for heparin use, ten for a combination of heparin and stockings, and lowest for a combination of intermittent pneumatic compression and stockings with only seven pulmonary embolism cases[150]. The costs of initial prophylaxis are roughly equivalent to the costs of later pulmonary embolism therapy, although most clinicians would view the former regimen more favorably in terms of patient benefit.

An issue of paramount importance to patients is the ability to communicate. The use of a visual communication board was studied by

Stovsky and co-workers[151] in 40 post-cardiothoracic surgery patients, with minimal improvement in satisfaction scales for patients and nurses. Clearly, the ability to speak with a tracheostomy in place is desirable, using a fenestrated tracheostomy tube, air-flow tube or one-way valve. Advantages to the patient include secretion reduction, speech capability, decreased aspiration and improved sense of smell associated with better appetite, which result in improvement in overall well-being.

OUTCOME MODELS

Perhaps the most commonly invoked and simplest outcome model involves the use of persistent organ failure criteria to predict outcome. Knaus and colleagues[152] analyzed 5677 consecutive general surgery ICU admissions and found that failure of a single organ system persisting for at least 48 h resulted in up to 40% mortality, which increased to 60% with failure of two systems and up to 98% of patients not surviving an ICU stay if failure of three systems occurred. There is a progressive linear increase in mortality with increase of the number of organ systems involved, from a baseline of no systems (1% mortality) to seven systems associated with 86% mortality (Table 3)[152–154].

Similar analyses of 203 patients by Crump and associates[153] and 1136 surgical patients by Darling and co-workers[154] suggested that another important consideration is the specific organ system involved. The

Table 3 Outcome associated with organ system failure in surgical patients. Data from references 152–154

	Mortality (%)	
Number of organ systems	*Absolute or range*	*Cumulative*
0	1	
1	13–40	26
2	34–60	47
3	45–98	73
4	83–93	88
5	68	
6	96	
7	86	

pulmonary system was most commonly affected in surgical (78%) and trauma (83%) patients (Table 4)[153,154]. Persistent cardiovascular system involvement resulted in the most significant mortality rate, found in 79% of surgical patients and 100% of trauma patients[153,154].

Manship and colleagues[155] evaluated multisystem organ failure in a group of 77 SICU patients, identifying mortality due to sepsis in 44 (58%), followed by respiratory failure (13%), refractory shock (10%), liver failure (10%) and myocardial infarction in 9% of patients. The development of sepsis and subsequent mortality in this study correlated with poor nutritional status, diabetes mellitus, use of steroids, splenectomy and a total lymphocyte count of less than 700 cells/mm^3.

A multivariate analysis of 538 ICU patients with multisystem organ failure was performed by Tran and co-workers[156], reporting a 16% (88 of 538) incidence associated with 52% mortality. Multiple logistic regression identified age, malnutrition, APACHE II score and multisystem organ failure score as predictors of mortality[156]. Proprietary outcome prediction models are outlined in Table 5[35,157-172].

The Glasgow outcome scale (GOS) provides a descriptive analysis of functional outcome in patients with primary or secondary cerebral injury[157]. The therapeutic intervention scoring system (TISS) grades the utility of 57 ICU interventions and evaluates the efficacy of personnel, equipment, resource utilization and staffing[158]. The TISS 1983 update increased the analysis to 76 ICU therapeutic maneuvers, graded on a 1–4 scale with only the maximal score for like interventions included[159]. Regression analysis using the $y = 0.5 + 1.03x$ relationship reveals a similar line of identity for both the 1974 and 1983 scoring systems[158,159].

Table 4 Specific organ system involvement in surgical patients. Data from references 153 and 154

Organ system	Incidence (%)		Mortality (%)	
	Range	*Cumulative*	*Range*	*Cumulative*
Cardiovascular	11–84	47	70–89	79
Hematological	17–45	31	56–86	71
Renal	44–63	53	69–74	71
Gastrointestinal	22–27	24	39–72	55
Hepatic	21–50	35	64–65	64
Central nervous system	39–86	62	47–69	58
Pulmonary	74–83	78	50–63	56

Table 5 Outcome prediction model. Data from references 35 and 157–172

Method	Variables	Scale	Range	Monitor	Prediction				
					Accuracy (%)	Sensitivity (%)	Specificity (%)	Positive predictive value (%)	Negative predictive value (%)
Glasgow outcome scale (GOS)	1, death; 2, persistent vegetative state; 3, severe disability; 4, moderate disability; 5, good recovery	0–5	0–5	functional outcome					
Therapeutic intervention scoring system (TISS)	57 ICU interventions; 1, active transplant; 2, ICU personnel; 3, ICU technology; 4, standard code	1–4	0–70	resource staffing budget		96	95		
Acute physiology and chronic health evaluation (APACHE) system	I: 4 health indicators 34 physiological variables	0–4	0–50	survival	81	97	49	90	79
	II: age, general health, 12 physiological variables	0–4	0–71	survival	86	47	95	69	88
	III: age, comorbid conditions, 20 physiological variables	0–24 0–23	0–299 0–252	predictive equation	88	50	96	73	90

Table 5 Continued over

Table 5 *Continued*

Method	Variables	Scale	Range	Monitor	Prediction			Positive predictive value (%)	Negative predictive value (%)
					Accuracy (%)	Sensitivity (%)	Specificity (%)		
Simplified acute physiology score (SAPS)	I: 14 physiological variables II: 17 variables, age, chronic health, admission	0–4	0–56 0–163	mortality		69 (0.883, GOF)	69 (0.88, ROC)		
Multiple logistic regression (MLR) model	7 variables, age, systolic pressure, number of organ systems, infection, type of admission, level of consciousness, cancer			regression	87	50	96	75	89
Mortality prediction model (MPM)	OT: 7 variables II: 15 variables	0–1 0–1		mortality	80 (0.623, GOF)	59 (0.837, ROC)	90	74	82

ICU, intensive care unit; GOF, goodness of fit; ROC, receiver operating characteristic; OT, over time

The current outcome prediction standard is the acute physiology and chronic health evaluation (APACHE) system, examining the patient's age and premorbid condition, combined with illness variables. APACHE I evaluated 805 ICU admissions and classified health status and physiological variables to achieve an 81% accuracy of prediction[160].

The basis of this prediction tool is the chronic health evaluation, in which patients are classified as category A with prior good health, B with mild to moderate limitation of activity, C with serious but not incapacitating restriction of activity, and D if bedridden or institution-alized as a result of illness, combined with the acute physiology score (APS) where 34 variables are graded on a 0–4 scale (APS-34)[160]. The APS for the above patient group was a mean of 15 with a range of 0–50, with each additional point increasing hospital mortality by 2%[160].

Univariate logistic regression analysis suggests an inverse correlation between either chronic health status or physiology score and survival, while multiple logistic regression analysis suggests the overwhelming significance of the physiology score with only class D health status affecting outcome[160].

APACHE I analysis of this study sample demonstrated good sensitivity (97%) and positive predictive value (90%), indicating that those who were predicted to survive at a level of 0.50 predicted risk did so. However, the specificity (49%) and negative predictive value (79%) were poor, indicating that some of those who were predicted to die actually survived[160]. Further validation studies were then suggested (Table 6).

APACHE II evaluated 5815 ICU admissions, adding an age criterion and decreasing the significance of physiological variables measured from 34 to 12 (APS-12) to achieve 86% accuracy[35]. This prediction model was constructed on the hypothesis that the severity of acute disease can be measured by quantifying the degree of abnormality of multiple physiological variables[35]. However, this version refined the baseline chronic health and age components in an attempt to improve specificity. APACHE II classification of outcome for 0.50 predicted risk demon-strated decreased sensitivity (47%) with adequate positive predictive value (69.6%), while the specificity (94.9%) and negative predictive value (87.9%) were improved[35]. Thus, APACHE II offered a simpler approach to classification of physiological abnormality, requiring an accurate description of acute and chronic disease to predict survival.

Comparison of APACHE II with physicians' prediction of outcome using receiver operating characteristic (ROC) curves suggests that the

Table 6 Survival prediction model*

	Model	Example
Predicted survival		
observed survival	TP	800
observed mortality	FP	200
Predicted mortality		
observed survival	FN	50
observed mortality	TN	100
Sensitivity (%)	$100 \times \dfrac{TP}{TP + FN}$	$100 \times \dfrac{800}{800 + 50} = 94.1$
Positive predictive value (%)	$100 \times \dfrac{TP}{TP + FP}$	$100 \times \dfrac{800}{800 + 200} = 80$
Specificity (%)	$100 \times \dfrac{TN}{TN + FP}$	$100 \times \dfrac{100}{100 + 200} = 33.3$
Negative predictive value (%)	$100 \times \dfrac{TN}{TN + FN}$	$100 \times \dfrac{100}{100 + 50} = 66.6$

*Sensitivity: probability that model will predict survival, when survival occurs; positive predictive value: proportion of individuals that survived, when survival was predicted by model; specificity: probability that model will predict mortality, when mortality occurs; negative predictive value: proportion of individuals that died, when mortality was predicted by model; predicted risk 0.5; TP, true positives; FP, false positives; FN, false negatives; TN, true negatives

physicians' (0.899) impressions were significantly better than APACHE II (0.796) predictions[161]. However, use of the APACHE II system was better for the less severely ill patient with a mortality risk of less than 30%[161]. Another area of concern is that APACHE II significantly underestimated mortality for patients admitted to the ICU from the floor (38% vs. 55%), from intermediate care (32% vs. 59%) and after interhospital transfer (21% vs. 36%), but was a good predictor of mortality in those patients admitted from the emergency department (25% vs. 22%)[162].

The current standard, APACHE III, was based on a study of 17 440 ICU patients, using age, comorbid illness and physiological variables in a predictive equation model to achieve 95% classification accuracy within 24 h of admission, where the risk estimate for hospital death was within 3% of those observed[163]. The major disease diagnostic category predicts regression coefficients for 78 medical–surgical non-operative and postoperative disease categories, as well as incorporating data based on the preadmission location (emergency department, ward, other hospital, other ICU and ICU readmission) of medical cases and an emergency qualifier for operative cases (Table 7)[35,160,163].

APACHE III performed reasonably well, with again better specificity (96.3%) and negative predictive value (90.2%) than sensitivity (50.4%) and positive predictive value (72.7%) within 24 h at a 0.50 predicted risk of hospital death[163]. The overall predictive accuracy was 88.1%, with 95% of ICU patients assigned a risk estimate within 3% of that actually observed[163]. However, this system is largely computer based and applicable to the retrospective analysis of group mortality using proprietary regression coefficients, as opposed to the prospective prediction of individual mortality.

APACHE III has been validated by other investigators, including Barie and colleagues in a group of 854 ICU patients, suggesting that selective underestimation of mortality found in APACHE II had been remedied[164]. Areas of improvement include in those with traumatic injury, specifically severe head injury.

The simplified acute physiology score (SAPS) grades 14 biological and clinical variables on a 0–4 scale, validated in a population of 679 medical (60%) and surgical (40%) patients[166]. There was a linear increase in mortality as the SAPS increased from 4 (10.7%) to 21 or greater (81.1%), comparing favorably with the APS and yielding a similar ROC curve[165]. Thus, this scoring system attempts to offer acceptable sensitivity and specificity without the complexity of assessing prior health status or individual disease conditions.

The multiple logistic regression (MLR) model uses seven independent admission variables, disease indicators and dependent treatment variables derived from a group of 755 patient admissions, to achieve 87% accuracy (Table 8)[166]. This model first used a linear discriminant function analysis with forward stepping to delineate those univariate variables that are different in patients who die or survive to discharge[166,167]. The probability of mortality Pr $(y = 1)$ for the individual patient is dependent on condition and treatment variables $(X_1, X_2...X_k)$, which are considered sequentially by a multivariate technique, eliminating those that are not correlated with survival[166,168]. The model uses estimated logistic coefficients B, standard error (SE), adjusted odds ratio (OR) and 95% confidence interval (CI) for the odds ratio, which estimates the likelihood of mortality if the variable is present[166].

113

Table 7 Probability of mortality using acute physiology and chronic health evaluation (APACHE) system: APACHE III reference data. Data from references 35, 160 and 163

Data	Points
Age (years)	
≤ 44	0
45–59	5
60–64	11
65–69	13
70–74	16
75–84	17
≥ 85	24
Comorbid conditions	
AIDS	23
Hepatic failure	16
Lymphoma	13
Metastatic cancer	11
Leukemia/multiple myeloma	10
Immunosuppression	15
Cirrhosis	4
Acute physiology data	
Pulse (beats/min)	0–17
Mean blood pressure (mmHg)	0–23
Temperature (°C)	0–20
Respiratory rate (breaths/min)	0–18
pao_2 (mmHg)	0–15
Alveolar-arterial oxygen gradient (A-aDo_2; mmHg)	0–14
Hematocrit (%)	0–3
White blood cell count (10^3/mm^3)	0–19
Creatinine (mg/dl)	
acute renal failure (ARF)	0–7
chronic renal failure (CRF)	0–10
Urine output (ml/day)	0–15
Blood urea nitrogen (mg/dl)	0–12
Sodium (mmol/l)	0–4
Albumin (g/dl)	0–11
Bilirubin (mg/dl)	0–16
Glucose (mg/dl)	0–9

Table 7   Continued

Table 7 *Continued*

Data	Points
pH	0–12
Neurological	0–48

Major disease categories
Non-operative
Postoperative

Multiple logistic regression equation, binary dichotomous outcome model

$$\ln \times \frac{R}{1 - R} = A + B_i X_i$$

where ln is natural log of risk of mortality, R is risk of mortality, $R/(1 - R)$ is the odds of death, A is the estimated intercept and B is the estimated coefficient for each independent variable X

The MLR-1985 model demonstrated a sensitivity of 50% and a positive predictive value of 75%, while the specificity of 96% and negative predictive value of 89% resulted in an 87% rate of correct classification for mortality[166]. This method was suggested to provide reasonable accuracy in predicting mortality by analyzing a limited number of variables.

The mortality prediction model (MPM-1988) modified the regression equation to include surgical observations at admission, 24 h and 48 h to predict mortality in a 2783-patient group[169]. The cumulative risk of mortality is the MPM_{OT} 'over time', where X_1 is the mortality risk at admission (MPM_0), X_2 is estimated at 24 h (MPM_0–MPM_{24}) and X_3 is estimated at 48 h (MPM_{24}–MPM_{48}) with incorporation of survival contingency (Table 9)[169]. The sensitivity (58.7%) and positive predictive value (74.0%) are reasonable, while the specificity (90.2%) and negative predictive value (82.2%) are superior to those resulting from the use of MPM_0 alone[169]. Thus, the overall classification of mortality (MPM_{OT}) achieves an 80.1% rate of correct classification, slightly improved over the admission mortality prediction rate (MPM_0) of 76.7%[169].

Lemeshow and colleagues'[170] mortality prediction model was then validated in a 1997-patient group (MPM_{0CPR} where CPR is cardiopulmonary resuscitation prior to admission) with an excellent goodness of fit or correspondence between observed and expected deaths within

115

Table 8 Probability of mortality using multiple logistic regression (MLR) model or mortality probability model I (MPM I): mean regression coefficients. Table adapted from reference 166

Variable	*No (0)*	*Yes (1)*	MLR_0 $\bar{B}$	MLR_0 $SE(\bar{B})$	MLR_{24} $\bar{B}$	MLR_{24} $SE(\bar{B})$
Constant	—	—	-3.000	1.500	-5.930	0.779
Level of consciousness	—	coma	2.630	0.464	4.53	1.110
Type of admission	elective	emergency	1.630	0.410	0.928	0.414
Cancer	—	present	1.490	0.444		
Infection	—	probable	0.677	0.251	1.310	0.297
Number of organ failures	0	OR 1	0.595	0.121	0.336	0.150
Age (10-year OR)	—	OR 10 years	0.038	0.007	0.038	0.009
Systolic blood pressure (mmHg)	—	low	0.048	0.019		
SBP^2		high	0.000131	0.00007		
Inspired oxygen fraction	—				1.170	0.424
Shock	—				0.998	0.328

$$Pr(y = 1 \, X_1, X_2 \ldots X_k) = \frac{e^{(B_0 + B_1X_1 + B_2X_2 + \ldots B_kX_k)}}{1 + e^{(B_0 + B_1X_1 + B_2X_2 + \ldots B_kX_k)}}$$

where *Pr* is the probability of mortality, (y = 1) or survival (y = 0), *X* is a variable and *B* is a coefficient.
Example: a 65-year-old comatose patient with lung cancer presented as an emergency case with pneumonia, renal failure and hypotension (blood pressure 60 mmHg):

Table 8 Continued

Table 8 *Continued*

Variable	No (0)	Yes (1)	MLR_0		MLR_{24}	
			B	$SE(B)$	B	$SE(B)$

Pr (mortality $1X_1, X_2, ..., X_k$)

$B = [[-3.000) + (2.630) + (1.630) + (1.490) + (0.677) + (3 \times 0.595) + (65 \times 0.038) + (60 \times 0.048) + (3600 \times 0.000\ 13)]$

$= 3.427 + 1.79 + 2.47 + (-2.88) + 0.4680$

$= 5.2750$

$Pr = \dfrac{e^{4.0836}}{1 + e^{4.0836}} = \dfrac{195.3905}{1 + 195.3905} = 0.9949$

Probability of mortality is 99.5%

OR, odds ratio; SE, standard error

Table 9 Probability of mortality using mortality prediction model 'over time' (MPM$_{OT}$): regression coefficients. Table adapted from reference 169

Variable	No (0)	Yes (1)	MPM_0	MPM_{24}	MPM_{48}
Constant	—	—	-2.9678	-6.5917	-5.8601
Level of consciousness	—	coma	2.8902	3.4986	2.8644
Type of admission	elective	emergency	1.2671	0.80224	0.9602
CPR prior to admission	—	present	1.0137		
Cancer	—	present	0.94131	0.99476	0.8155
Chronic renal failure	—	yes	0.64049		
Infection	—	probable	0.55592	0.53755	0.47138
Age (10-year relative risk)			0.047789	0.044142	0.042383
ICU admission (≤ 6 months)				0.43946	
Heart rate (10-beat relative risk)				0.06736	
Surgical service				-0.37987	-0.70808
Systolic blood pressure				-0.04591	
SBP^2				0.000116	
Prothrombin time >3 s above normal				0.73764	0.90928
Probable shock				0.67367	
Urine output <150 ml in any 8 h				0.65128	0.99015
Hypoxia (pO_2 <60 torr)				0.49666	0.81206
C(a-v)O$_2$ gradient (FiO$_2$ >0.5)				0.47462	
Creatinine >2.0 mg/dl				0.45716	

Table 9 Continued

Table 9 *Continued*

Variable	No (0)	Yes (1)	B		
			MPM_0	MPM_{24}	MPM_{48}
Hours of mechanical ventilation				0.026336	0.021409
Number of lines (1-line relative risk)				0.15376	0.017262
Total hours of vasoactive drug therapy					

$$Pr(y) = \frac{e^{logit}}{1 + e^{logit}}$$

where $Pr(y)$ is the probability of mortality over time, y is the discharge status and
$logit = \bar{B}_0 + \bar{B}_1X_1 + \bar{B}_2X_2 + \ldots + \bar{B}_kX_k$ where X is a variable, B is a coefficient.

Example: a patient has an admission prediction of mortality of 75%, followed by 50% at 24 h and 25% at 48 h. Using the following regression coefficients: constant, −2.9287; MPM_0, 6.3373; MPM_0–MPM_{24}, −5.1914; MPM_{24}–MPM_{48}, −3.0546:

$$
\begin{aligned}
MPM_{OT} &= \text{constant} + B_1X_1\,(MPM_0) + B_2X_2\,(MPM_0\!-\!MPM_{24}) + B_3X_3\,(MPM_{24}\!-\!MPM_{48}) \\
&= -2.9287 + 6.3373\,(0.75) + [-5.1914\,(0.75\!-\!0.50)] + [-3.0546\,(0.50\!-\!0.25)] \\
&= -2.9287 + 4.7529 + (-1.2978) + (-0.7636) \\
&= -0.2372
\end{aligned}
$$

$$Pr(y) = \frac{e^{-0.2372}}{1 + e^{-0.2372}} = \frac{0.7887}{1.7887} = 0.4409$$

Probability of mortality over time is 44.1%

CPR, cardiopulmonary resuscitation; ICU, intensive care unit

119

risk categories ($p = 0.74$), and correct classification with 86.1% accuracy. However, Le Gall and co-workers' SAPS system demonstrated the best specificity (97.0%) and predictive value for mortality (87.7%), while Knaus and associates' APS system demonstrated the highest sensitivity (58.8%) and predictive value for surviving (90.2%)[35].

The mortality probability models (MPM II) evaluated 19 124 patients using both a predictive component (MPM_0) and a quality assurance component (MPM_{24}) (Table 10)[171]. The admission model (MPM_0) analyzed 15 variables and calibrated well, showing goodness of fit ($p = 0.623$) between observed and predicted results, and discriminated well, showing an area under the ROC curve of 0.837[171]. Likewise, the MPM_{24} contained five admission and eight hospital variables, calibrating well ($p = 0.764$) and discriminating well (area under the ROC curve 0.844)[171]. Thus, this version of the predictive model analyzes the admission and 24-h MPM scores independently.

The SAPS II evaluated 13 152 patients to establish a subjective model based on included variables, in contrast with the more objective measures such as the APACHE and MPM scores where regression coefficients are derived (Table 11)[172]. This model examined 17 variables, including 12 physiological measures, age, type of admission (scheduled or unscheduled surgical, medical) and presence of chronic disease (AIDS, metastatic cancer, hematological malignancy)[172]. The goodness of fit ($p = 0.883$, $p = 0.104$) and areas under the ROC curve (0.88, 0.86) were acceptable for the developmental and validation samples, respectively[172-174]. The SAPS II is an easily performed method examining a small number of variables, providing reasonable mortality prediction capacity without a specific disease category.

Lemeshow and Jean-Roger's comparison of the currently available outcome prediction models[175] observes that APACHE III and SAPS II grade the worst value on the day of admission, MPM II allows grading at four times (0, 24, 48, 72 h) and APACHE III requires proprietary information for outcome prediction. The goodness of fit was excellent for SAPS II and MPM II while this was not reported for APACHE III, and the areas under the ROC curve were good for all models studied.

Physicians are better at predicting survival (87%) than mortality (41%), and are correct in 58–73% of cases in predicting long-term nursing care requirements[176]. Therefore, subjective physicians' impressions concerning patient mortality are often successful at a rate less than chance. Christensen and colleagues[177] compared physician with APACHE

Table 10 Probability of mortality using mortality probability model II (MPM II): regression coefficients. Table adapted from reference 171

Variable	MPM_0 B	MPM_{24}
Constant	−5.46836	−5.64592
Physiology		
Coma	1.48592	
Heart rate ≥ 150 beats/min	0.45603	
Systolic blood pressure < 90 mmHg	1.06127	
Chronic diagnosis		
Chronic renal insufficiency	0.91906	
Cirrhosis	1.13681	
Metastatic neoplasm	1.19979	
Acute diagnosis		
Acute renal failure	1.48210	
Cardiac dysrhythmia	0.28095	
Cerebrovascular incident	0.21338	
Gastrointestinal bleeding	0.39653	
Intracranial mass effect	0.86533	
Other		
Age (10-year odds ratio)	0.03057	
Cardiopulmonary resuscitation	0.56995	
Mechanical ventilation	0.79105	
Non-elective surgery	1.19098	
Variables ascertained at admission		
Age (10-year odds ratio)		0.03268
Cirrhosis		1.08745
Intracranial mass effect		0.91314
Metastatic neoplasm		1.16109
Medical or unscheduled surgery admission		0.83404
24-h assessments		
Coma or stupor		1.68790
Creatinine ≥ 2.0 mg/dl		0.72283
Confirmed infection		0.49742
Mechanical ventilation		0.80845

Table 10   Continued over

121

Table 10   *Continued*

Variable	MPM_0 B	MPM_{24}
$pO_2 < 60$ mmHg		0.46677
Prothrombin time > 3 s above normal		0.55352
Urine output < 150 ml/hr		0.82286
Vasoactive drugs ≥ 1 h		0.71628

$$Pr \text{ (hospital mortality)} = \frac{e^{g(x)}}{1 + e^{g(x)}}$$

where *Pr* is the probability of mortality, $g(x) = B_0 + B_1X_1 + B_2X_2 + \dots + B_kX_k$, *X* is a variable and *B* is a coefficient.

Example: a 65-year-old comatose patient with lung cancer presented as an emergency case with pneumonia, renal failure and hypotension (blood pressure 60 mmHg):

Pr (mortality $1X_1, X_2, \dots X_k$)

B = constant (−5.46836) + age (65 × 0.03057) + coma (1.48592) + metastatic neoplasm (1.19979) + renal failure (1.48210) + systolic blood pressure (1.06127)

   = 1.74362

$$Pr = \frac{e^{1.7436}}{1 + e^{1.7436}} = \frac{5.7178}{1 + 5.7178} = 0.8511$$

Probability of mortality is 85.1%

II predictions and suggested that physicians were good predictors but slightly pessimistic, predicting survival in 40–70% of cases in relation to 72% observed survival. Also, the level of training correlated with forecasting accuracy, with attending physicians scoring better than residents, followed by interns, while fellows and nurses significantly underestimated survival[177].

OUTCOME AND QUALITY OF LIFE

The average mortality rate for surgical ICU patients is 13% (range 7–24%) from grouped series of 8292 representative patients[97,167,178,179].

Table 11 Probability of mortality using simplified acute physiology score (SAPS II). Table adapted from reference 172

Variable	Lower limit		Upper limit	
	Value	*Score*	*Value*	*Score*
Age (years)	<40	0	>80	18
Heart rate (beats/min)	<40	11	≥160	7
Systolic blood pressure (mmHg)	<70	13	≥200	2
Body temperature (°C)	<39	0	≥39	3
Ventilation or pulmonary artery pressure monitoring				
PaO_2 mmHg/FiO_2	<100	11	≥200	6
Urinary output (l/day)	<0.5	11	≥1.0	0
Serum urea level (mg/dl)	<28	0	≥84	10
White blood cell count (× 10^3/mm^3)	<10	12	≥20.0	3
Potassium (mmol/d)	<3.0	3	≥5.0	3
Sodium (mmol/l)	<125	5	≥145	1
Bicarbonate (mEq/l)	<15	6	≥20	0
Bilirubin (mg/dl)	<4.0	0	≥6.0	9
Glasgow coma score	<6	26	14–15	0
Chronic diseases	metastatic cancer	9	hematological malignancy	10
			AIDS	17
			medical	6
Type of admission	scheduled surgical	0	unscheduled surgical	8

Table 11 Continued over

123

Table 11 *Continued*

	Lower limit		Upper limit	
Variable	*Value*	*Score*	*Value*	*Score*

$$Pr\ (y = 1/\text{logit}) = \frac{e^{\text{logit}}}{1 + e^{\text{logit}}}$$

where $Pr\ (y = 1/\text{logit})$ is the probability of mortality and logit $= B_0 + B_1\ (\text{SAPS II}) + B_2\ [\ln\ (\text{SAPS II} + 1)] = -7.7361 + 0.0737\ (\text{SAPS II}) + 0.9971\ [\ln\ (\text{SAPS II} + 1)]$, where B is a coefficient.

Example: a 65-year-old comatose patient with lung cancer presented emergently with pneumonia, renal failure and hypotension (blood pressure <60 mmHg):

Sum = age (12) + systolic blood pressure (13) + malignancy (9) + medical (6) = 40

Logit = $-7.7631 + 0.0737\ (40) + 0.9971\ [\ln\ (41)]$

$= -7.7631 + 2.948 + 3.7028$

$= -1.112$

$Pr\ (y = 1/\text{logit}) = \dfrac{e^{-1.112}}{1 + e^{-1.112}} = \dfrac{0.3288}{1 + 0.3288} = 0.2474$

Probability of mortality is 24.7%

124

Zimmerman and co-workers' evaluation of ICU mortality suggested that the 12% ICU rate compared favorably with the 20% incidence of mortality found on the general ward[179].

Patients that survive their ICU course incur a 3.4-fold increase in mortality during the first year after discharge, which equilibrates to the normal cohort at 4 years post-discharge, according to Ridley and Plenderleith[180]. In another study, those patients who underwent long-term (more than 30 days) ICU care had a 39% hospital mortality rate, 31% were discharged to another health-care facility and 50% eventually returned home[181]. The incidence of patients requiring prolonged ICU care was 1.2% (223 of 18 126), but these patients had additional sequelae with a 50% 1-year mortality rate[181]. However, 30% of those returning home were able to function independently.

Quality of life should be a paramount issue for patients' families and physicians. Miranda and Miranda[178] performed retrospective interviews of 273 patients suffering a 24.5–35% rate of mortality for those over 65 years. Of the 97 survivors, 40 (41%) reported that they were satisfied with their outcome in performing their normal routine, while 57 (59%) were unhappy with their rehabilitation end-point[178]. However, Chelluri and colleagues[45] reported a similar study in the elderly, and found that most patients were happy with their ICU course and outcome and, most importantly, would undergo the same care again in a hypothetical scenario[45].

CONCLUSION

The morbidity and mortality encountered in taking care of the critically ill patient are inevitable. Complications can be minimized, however, using a dedicated practitioner who combines the expertise of medicine, anesthesia, surgery, pediatrics and emergency medicine disciplines. The intensivist seeks to optimize preoperative assessment and postoperative care consistent with patient and family needs, to achieve the best possible outcome for the ICU patient.

REFERENCES

1. Satter P. Surgical intensive care. *Zentralbl Chir* 1977;102:321–5

2. Elver MS, Ali MK. Surgical treatment of the cancer patient: pre-operative assessment and perioperative medical management. *J Surg Oncol* 1990;44:185–90

3. Trask AL, Faber DR. The intensive care unit – who's in charge? The private practice view. *Arch Surg* 1990;125:1105–8

4. Frey P. Respiratory failure and surgery [in Germany]. *Schweiz Med Wochenschr* 1979;109:1562–4

5. Davies JM, Strunin L. Anesthesia in 1984: how safe is it? *Can Med Assoc J* 1984;131:437–41

6. Wylie WD. 'There, but for the grace of God…'. *Ann R Coll Surg Engl* 1975;56:171–80

7. Saklad M. Grading of patients for surgical procedures. *Anesthesiology* 1941;2:281–4

8. Dripps RD, Lamont A, Eckenhoff JE, *et al.* The role of anesthesia in surgical mortality. *J Am Med Assoc* 1961;178:261–6

9. House of Delegates. New classification of physical status. *Anesthesiology* 1963;24:111

10. Goldman L, Caldera DL, Nussbaum SR, *et al.* Multifactorial index of cardiac risk in noncardiac surgical procedures. *N Engl J Med* 1977;297:845–50

11. Zeldin RA, Math B. Assessing cardiac risk in patients who undergo noncardiac surgical procedures. *Can J Surg* 1984;27:402–4

12. Detsky AS, Abrams HB, McLaughlin JR, *et al.* Predicting cardiac complications in patients undergoing non-cardiac surgery. *J Gen Intern Med* 1986;1:211–19

13. Holdcroft A. Outpatient preoperative assessment: the anaesthetist's view. *Ann R Coll Surg Engl* 1980;62:382–5

14. Sanders DP, McKinney FW, Harris WH. Clinical evaluation and cost effectiveness of preoperative laboratory assessment on patients undergoing total hip arthroplasty. *Orthopedics* 1989;12:1449–53

15. Mangano DT, Siliciano D, Hollenberg M, *et al.* Postoperative myocardial ischemia. Therapeutic trials using intensive analgesia following surgery. *Anesthesiology* 1992;76:342–53

16. Kirsch JR, Diringer MN, Borel CO, *et al.* Preoperative lumbar epidural morphine improves postoperative analgesia and ventilatory function after transsternal thymectomy in patients with myasthenia gravis. *Crit Care Med* 1991;19:1474–9

17. Greenburg AG, Saik RP, Farris JM, *et al.* Operative mortality in general surgery. *Am J Surg* 1982;144:22–8

18. Luft HS, Bunker JP, Enthoven AC. Should operations be regionalized? The empirical relation between surgical volume and mortality. *N Engl J Med* 1979;301:1364–9

19. Flood NB, Scott WR, Ewy W. Does practice make perfect? Part I: The relation between hospital volume and outcomes for selected diagnostic categories. *Med Care* 1984;22:98–114

20. Sloan FA, Perrin JM, Valvona J. In-hospital mortality of surgical patients: is there an empiric basis for standard setting? *Surgery* 1986; 99:446–510

21. Hannan EL, O'Donnell JF, Kilburn H Jr, *et al*. Investigation of the relationship between volume and mortality for surgical procedures performed in New York state hospitals. *J Am Med Assoc* 1989;262:503–10

22. Lauven PM, Stoeckel H, Ebeling BJ. Perioperative morbidity and mortality of geriatric patients. A retrospective study of 3905 cases [in German]. *Anasth, Intensivther, Notfallmed* 1990;25:3–9

23. Crucitti F, Doglietto GB, Bellantone R, *et al*. Effects of surgical treatment in thymoma with myasthenia gravis: our experience in 103 patients. *J Surg Oncol* 1992;50:43–6

24. Okuyama A, Goda Y, Kawahigashi H, *et al*. Perioperative management for patients with hypertrophic cardiomyopathy undergoing non-cardiac surgery [in Japanese]. *Masui – Jpn J Anesthesiol* 1992;41:119–21

25. Cole RR, Cotton RT. Preventing postoperative complications in the adult cystic fibrosis patient. *Int J Pediatr Otorhinolaryngol* 1990;18:263–9

26. Reding R, Michel LA, Donckier J, *et al*. Surgery in patients on long-term steroid therapy: a tentative model for risk assessment. *Br J Surg* 1990;77:1175–8

27. Perilli V, Tacchino R, Sollazzi L, *et al*. Anesthesiological problems in the obese patient. Clinical experience in the treatment of 54 cases [in Italian]. *Minerva Anestesiol* 1991;57:389–94

28. Thibault GE, Mulley AG, Barnett GO, *et al*. Medical intensive care: interventions, and outcomes. *N Engl J Med* 1980;302:938–42

29. Mundt DJ, Gage RW, Lemeshow S, *et al*. Intensive care unit patient follow-up: mortality, functional status, and return to work at six months. *Arch Intern Med* 1989;149:68–72

30. Smith SL. Postoperative perfusion deficits. *Crit Care Nurs Clin North Am* 1990;2:567–78

31. Kockerling F, Gall FP. Intensive care of geriatric patients in surgery [in German]. *Fortschr Med* 1992;110:238–40

32. Frede KE, Lanter G. Surgical intensive care in advanced age [in German]. *Helv Chir Acta* 1991;57:903–7

33. Older P, Smith R. Experience with the preoperative invasive measurement of hemodynamic, respiratory and renal function in 100 elderly patients scheduled for major abdominal surgery. *Anaesth Intens Care* 1988;16:389–95

34. Brown JJ, Sullivan G. Effect on ICU mortality of a full-time critical care specialist. *Chest* 1989;96:127–9
35. Knaus WA, Draper EA, Wagner DP, *et al.* APACHE II: a severity of disease classification system. *Crit Care Med* 1985;13:818–29
36. Li TCM, Phillips MC, Shaw L, *et al.* On-site physician staffing in a community hospital intensive care unit. Impact on test and procedure use and on patient outcome. *J Am Med Assoc* 1984;252:2023–7
37. Reynolds HN, Haupt MT, Thill-Baharozian MC, *et al.* Impact of critical care physician staffing on patients with septic shock in a university hospital medical intensive care unit. *J Am Med Assoc* 1988; 260:3446–50
38. Hainer BL, Lawler FH. Comparison of critical care provided by family physicians and general internists. *J Am Med Assoc* 1988;260:354–8
39. Zimmerman JE, Shortell SM, Knaus WA, *et al.* Value and cost of teaching hospitals: a prospective multicenter, inception cohort study. *Crit Care Med* 1993;21:1432–42
40. Schrader LL, McMillen MA, Watson CB, *et al.* Is routine preoperative hemodynamic evaluation of nonagenarians necessary? *J Am Geriatr Soc* 1991;39:1–5
41. Del Guercio LR, Cohn JD. Monitoring operative risk in the elderly. *J Am Med Assoc* 1980;243:1350–5
42. Yamanaka H, Hiramatsu Y, Kojima Y, *et al.* Postoperative pulmonary complication and surgical treatment of esophageal cancer in aged patients – evaluation of preoperative risk factors and postoperative management [in Japanese]. *Nippon Kyobu Geka Gakkai Zasshi* 1991;39: 1055–61
43. Del Guercio LR, Savino JA, Morgan JC. Physiologic assessment of surgical diagnosis-related groups. *Ann Surg* 1985;202:519–23
44. Margulies DR, Lekawa ME, Bjerke HS, *et al.* Surgical intensive care in the nonagenarian. No basis for age discrimination. *Arch Surg* 1993; 128:753–6
45. Chelluri L, Pinsky MR, Donahoe M, *et al.* Long-term outcome of critically ill elderly patients requiring intensive care. *J Am Med Assoc* 1993; 269:3119–23
46. Berlauk JF, Abrams JH, Gilmour IJ, *et al.* Preoperative optimization of cardiovascular hemodynamics improves outcome in peripheral vascular surgery. A prospective, randomized clinical trial. *Ann Surg* 1991;214:289–97
47. Zimmerman JE, Shortell SM, Rousseau DM, *et al.* Improving intensive care: observations based on organizational case studies in nine intensive care units: a prospective, multicenter study. *Crit Care Med* 1993; 21:1443–51

48. Rapoport J, Teres D, Lemeshow S, *et al*. A method for assessing the clinical performance and cost-effectiveness of intensive care units: a multicenter inception cohort study. *Crit Care Med* 1994;22:1385–91

49. Goenen M, Jacquemart JL, Galvez S, *et al*. Preoperative left ventricular dysfunction and operative risks in coronary bypass surgery. *Chest* 1987;92:804–6

50. Gibbs HR, Swafford J, Nguyen HD, *et al*. Postoperative atrial fibrillation in cancer surgery: preoperative risks and clinical outcome. *J Surg Oncol* 1992;50:224–7

51. Steen PA, Tinker JH, Tarhan S. Myocardial reinfarction after anesthesia and surgery. *J Am Med Assoc* 1978;239:2566–70

52. Girardi LN, Barie PS. Improved survival after intraoperative cardiac arrest in noncardiac surgical patients. *Arch Surg* 1995;130:15–18

53. Sakata R, Funatsu H, Higuchi K, *et al*. Cardiac operation in patients older than 70 years [in Japanese]. *Nippon Kyobu Geka Gakkai Zasshi* 1991;92:1123–6

54. McClellan M, McNeil BJ, Newhouse JP. Does more intensive treatment of acute myocardial infarction in the elderly reduce mortality? *J Am Med Assoc* 1994;272:859–66

55. Cahalan MK, Litt L, Botvinick EH, *et al*. Advances in noninvasive cardiovascular imaging: implications for the anesthesiologist. *Anesthesiology* 1987;66:356–72

56. Kessler G, Enders I. Impedance cardiography following cardiac surgery [in German]. *Anaesth Reanim* 1989;14:227–33

57. Viossat J, Abbou CB, Farias C, *et al*. Value of echocardiography in heart surgery [in French]. *Arch Mal Coeur* 1984;77:682–8

58. Carreras F, Pons-Llado G, Borras X, *et al*. Non-invasive preoperative assessment of chronic valvular heart disease by Doppler ultrasound. *Eur Heart J* 1988;9:874–8

59. Eagle KA, Singer DE, Brewster DC, *et al*. Dipyridamole–thallium scanning in patients undergoing vascular surgery. Optimizing preoperative evaluation of cardiac risk. *J Am Med Assoc* 1987;257:2185–9

60. Raff W, Sialer G, von Segesser L, *et al*. Perioperative myocardial perfusion scintigraphy at rest with technetium 99m methoxy-isobutylisonitrile before and after coronary bypass operations. *Eur J Nucl Med* 1991;18:99–105

61. Caramella JP, Aliot E, Claude E. Anesthesia and cardiac pacing [in French]. *Ann Fr Anesth Reanim* 1988;7:309–19

62. Vukmir RB. Emergency cardiac pacing. *Am J Emerg Med* 1993;11:166–76

63. Vukmir RB. Cardiac arrythmia: II Therapy. *Am J Emerg Med* 1995;13:459–70

64. Arena V, Gerometta PS, Pompilio G, *et al*. Preoperative management and surgical therapy in complicated acute infective endocarditis: a 5-year experience. *Cardiovasc Surg* 1993;1:419–25

65. Elefteriades JA, Tolis G Jr, Levi E, *et al*. Coronary artery bypass grafting in severe left ventricular dysfunction: excellent survival with improved ejection fraction and functional state. *J Am Coll Cardiol* 1993; 22:1411–17

66. Hattler BG, Madia C, Johnson C, *et al*. Risk stratification using the Society of Thoracic Surgeons' program. *Ann Thorac Surg* 1994;58:348–52

67. Kollef MH, Wragge T, Pasque C. Determinants of mortality and multi-organ dysfunction in cardiac surgery patients requiring prolonged mechanical ventilation. *Chest* 1995;107:1395–400

68. Georgeson S, Coombs AT, Eckman MH. Prophylactic use of the intra-aortic balloon pump in high-risk cardiac patients undergoing non-cardiac surgery: a decision analytic view. *Am J Med* 1992;92:665–78

69. Adamson RM, Dembitsky WP, Reichman RT, *et al*. Mechanical support: assist or nemesis? *J Thorac Cardiovasc Surg* 1989;98:915–20

70. Mulcahy D, Fitzgerald M, Wright C, *et al*. Long term follow up of severely ill patients who underwent urgent cardiac transplantation. *Br Med J* 1993;306:98–101

71. Slinger PD. Anaesthesia for lung resection. *Can J Anaesth* 1990;37(4 pt 2):Sxv–Sxxxii

72. Ebner H, Siudkamp N, Wex P, *et al*. Selection and preoperative treatment of over-seventy-year-old patients undergoing thoracotomy. *Thorac Cardiovasc Surg* 1985;33:268–71

73. Gorback MS, Moon RE, Massey JM. Extubation after transsternal thymectomy for myasthenia gravis: a prospective analysis. *South Med J* 1991;84:701–6

74. Pastorino U, Valente M, Bedini V, *et al*. Effect of chronic cardio-pulmonary disease or survival after resection for stage Ia lung cancer. *Thorax* 1982;37:680–3

75. Milledge JS, Nunn JF. Criteria of fitness for anaesthesia in patients with chronic obstructive lung disease. *Br Med J* 1975;3:670–3

76. Cottrell JJ, Ferson PF. Preoperative assessment of the thoracic surgical patient. *Clin Chest Med* 1992;13:47–53

77. Kearnery DJ, Lee TH, Reilly JJ, *et al*. Assessment of operative risk in patients undergoing lung resection: importance of predicted pulmonary function. *Chest* 1994;105:753–9

78. Busch E, Verazin G, Antkowiak JG, *et al*. Pulmonary complications in patients undergoing thoracotomy for lung carcinoma. *Chest* 1994;105: 760–6

79. von Knorring J, Lepantalo M, Lindgren L, *et al.* Cardiac arrhythmias and myocardial ischemia after thoracotomy for lung cancer. *Ann Thorac Surg* 1992;53:642–7

80. Gracey DR, Naessens JM, Krishan I, *et al.* Hospital and posthospital survival in patients mechanically ventilated for more than 29 days. *Chest* 1992;101:211–14

81. Corwin HL, Sprague SM, DeLaria GA, *et al.* Acute renal failure associated with cardiac operations. A case–control study. *J Thorac Cardiovasc Surg* 1989;98:1107–12

82. Mukau L, Latimer RG. Acute hemodialysis in the surgical intensive care unit. *Am Surg* 1988;54:548–52

83. Druml W, Lax F, Grimm G, *et al.* Acute renal failure in the elderly. *Clin Nephrol* 1994;41:342–9

84. Platt JF, Marn CS, Baliga PK, *et al.* Renal dysfunction in hepatic disease. Early identification with renal duplex Doppler US in patients who undergo liver transplantation. *Radiology* 1992;183:801–6

85. Sadaghdar H, Chelluri L, Bowles S, *et al.* Outcome of renal transplant recipients in the ICU. *Chest* 1995;107:402–5

86. Norris SO, Provo B, Stotts NA. Physiology of wound healing and risk factors that impede the healing process. *AACN Clin Issues Crit Care Nurs* 1990;1:545–52

87. Fass J. Wound healing disorder in surgery of colorectal cancer – a multifactorial computer analysis [in German]. *Langenbecks Arch Chir* 1985;367:63–73

88. Ulicny KS Jr, Hiratzka LF, Williams RB, *et al.* Sternotomy infection: poor prediction by acute phase response and delayed hypersensitivity. *Ann Thorac Surg* 1990;50:949–58

89. Maki DG. The use of antiseptics for handwashing by medical personnel. *J Chemother* 1989;1(Suppl 1):3–11

90. Carrel T, Schmid ER, von Segesser L, *et al.* Preoperative assessment of the likelihood of infection of the lower respiratory tract after cardiac surgery. *Thorac Cardiovasc Surg* 1991;39:85–8

91. Konrad F, Wiedeck H, Kilian J, *et al.* Risk factors in nosocomial pneumonia in intensive care patients. A prospective study to identify high-risk patients [in German]. *Anaesthetist* 1991;40:483–90

92. Culver DH, Horan TC, Gaynes RP, *et al.* Surgical wound infection rates by wound class, operative procedure, and patient risk index. National Nosocomial Infections Surveillance System. *Am J Med* 1991; 91:152S–7S

93. Sinanan M, Maier RV, Carrico CJ. Laparotomy for intra-abdominal sepsis in patients in an intensive care unit. *Arch Surg* 1984;119:652–8

94. Hartenauer U, Thulig B, Diemer W, *et al.* Effect of selective flora suppression on colonization, infection, and mortality in critically ill patients: a one-year, prospective consecutive study. *Crit Care Med* 1991;19:463–73

95. Gastinne H, Wolff M, Delatour F, *et al.* A controlled trial in intensive care units of selective decontamination of the digestive tract with nonabsorbable antibiotics. *N Engl J Med* 1992;326:594–9

96. National Committee for the Evaluation of Centoxin. The French National Registry of HA-1A (Centoxin) in septic shock. A cohort study of 600 patients. *Arch Intern Med* 1994;154:2484–91

97. Le Gall JR, Lemeshow S, Leleu G, *et al.* Customized probability models for early severe sepsis in adult intensive care patients. Intensive Care Unit Scoring Group. *J Am Med Assoc* 1995;273:644–50

98. Gravero D, Reggio D, Regge D, *et al.* Acute biliary pancreatitis. Therapeutic approach [in Italian]. *Minerva Chir* 1991;46:1235–43

99. Obertop H, Bruining HA, Schattenkerk ME, *et al.* Operative approach to cancer of the head of the pancreas and the peri-ampullary region. *Br J Surg* 1982;69:573–6

100. Cornwell EE 3rd, Rodriguez A, Mirvis SE, *et al.* Acute acalculous cholecystitis in critically injured patients. Preoperative diagnostic imaging. *Ann Surg* 1989;210:52–5

101. Aabo K, Pedersen H, Bach F, *et al.* Surgical management of intestinal obstruction in the late course of malignant disease. *Acta Chir Scand* 1984;150:173–6

102. Sarr MG, Bulkley GB, Zuidema GD. Preoperative recognition of intestinal strangulation obstruction. Prospective evaluation of diagnostic capability. *Am J Surg* 1983;145:176–82

103. Harju EJ, Pessi TT. Massive resection of the small bowel. *Int Surg* 1987;72:25–9

104. Waclawiczek HW. Surgically treated mechanical ileus [in German]. *Langenbecks Arch Chir* 1987;370:37–52

105. Udien P, Jiborn H, Jonsson K. Influence of selective mesenteric arteriography on the outcome of emergency surgery for massive, lower gastrointestinal hemorrhage. A 15 year experience. *Dis Colon Rect* 1986;29:561–6

106. Garrison RN, Cryer HM, Howard DA. Clarification of risk factors for abdominal operations in patients with hepatic cirrhosis. *Ann Surg* 1984;199:648–55

107. Herrera Carranza M, Pierez Bernal JB, Camacho Larana P, *et al.* Postoperative care in portal hypertension surgery [in Spanish]. *Med Clin (Spain)* 1979;72:1–12

108. Takenaka K, Kanematsu T, Fukuzawa K, *et al*. Can hepatic failure after surgery for hepatocellular carcinoma in cirrhotic patients be prevented? *World J Surg* 1990;14:123–7

109. Cole DJ, Ferguson CM. Complications of hepatic resection for colorectal carcinoma metastasis. *Am Surg* 1992;58:88–91

110. Foco A, Giordano A, Passarelli E, *et al*. Postoperative treatment of liver injuries in the surgical intensive care unit [in Italian]. *Minerva Med* 1981;72:17–20

111. Rypins EB, Sarfeh IJ, Collins-Irby D, *et al*. Asymptomatic peptic disease in patients undergoing major elective operations: a prospective endoscopic study. *Am J Gastroenterol* 1988;83:927–9

112. Cook DJ, Witt LG, Cook RJ, *et al*. Stress ulcer prophylaxis in the critically ill: a meta-analysis. *Am J Med* 1991;91:519–27

113. Byyny RL. Management of diabetics during surgery. *Post Grad Med* 1980;68:191–6

114. Romanchishen AF. Emergency and urgent operations in the treatment of patients with thyroid cancer [in Russian]. *Vopr Onkol* 1988;34:1088–92

115. Siebers MJ, Drinka PJ, Vergauwen C. Hyperthyroidism as a cause of atrial fibrillation in long-term care. *Arch Intern Med* 1992;152:2063–4

116. Pandya K, Lai C, Scheinhorn D, *et al*. Hypothyroidism and ventilator dependency. *Arch Intern Med* 1989;149:2115–16

117. Dahlberg PJ, Goellner MH, Pehling GB. Adrenal insufficiency secondary to adrenal hemorrhage: two case reports and a review of cases confirmed by computed tomography. *Arch Intern Med* 1990;150:905–9

118. Szalados JE, Vukmir RB. Acute adrenal insufficiency resulting from adrenal hemorrhage as indicated by post-operative hypotension. *Intens Care Med* 1994;20:216–18

119. Wong DH. Perioperative stroke. Part I: General surgery, carotid artery disease, and carotid endarterectomy. *Can J Anaesth* 1991;38:347–73

120. Mravinac CM. Neurological dysfunctions following cardiac surgery. *Crit Care Nurs Clin North Am* 1991;3:691–8

121. Nau HE, Hess W, Pohlen G, *et al*. Evoked potentials in intracranial operations: current status and our experiences [in German]. *Anaesthetist* 1987;36:116–25

122. Cellerin L, Ordronneau J, Chollet S, *et al*. Prognostic factors in the survival of patients with neuromuscular diseases after an episode of acute respiratory insufficiency [in French]. *Rev Mal Resp* 1994;11:263–70

123. Office of Medical Applications of Research. Perioperative red blood cell transfusion. *J Am Med Assoc* 1988;260:2700–3

124. Griffin KB. Postoperative bleeding. Current nursing management. *Crit Care Nurs Clin North Am* 1990;2:549–57

125. Loop FD, Higgins TL, Panda R, *et al.* Myocardial protection during cardiac operations. Decreased morbidity and lower cost with blood cardioplegia and coronary sinus perfusion. *J Thorac Cardiovasc Surg* 1992;104:608–18

126. Lorentz A, Osswald PM, Schilling M, *et al.* A comparison of auto-logous transfusion procedures in hip surgery [in German]. *Anaesthetist* 1991;40:205–13

127. The Veterans' Affairs Total Parenteral Nutrition Cooperative Study Group. Perioperative total parenteral nutrition in surgical patients. *N Engl J Med* 1991;325:525–32

128. Detsky AS, Baker JP, O'Rourke K, *et al.* Perioperative parenteral nutrition: a meta-analysis. *Ann Intern Med* 1987;107:195–203

129. Brown R, Bancewicz J, Hamid J, *et al.* Failure of delayed hyper-sensitivity skin testing to predict postoperative sepsis and mortality. *Br Med J* 1982;284:851–3

130. Dieckelmann A, Haupts M, Kaliwoda A, *et al.* Acute postoperative psychosyndromes. A prospective study and multivariate analysis of risk factors [in German]. *Chirurgia Klinik* 1989;60:470–4

131. McIntosh TK, Bush HL, Yeston NS, *et al.* Beta-endorphin, cortisol and postoperative delirium: a preliminary report. *Psychoneuroendocrinology* 1984;10:303–13

132. Sveinsson IS. Postoperative psychosis after heart surgery. *J Thorac Cardiovasc Surg* 1975;70:717–26

133. Savageau JA, Stanton BA, Jenkins CD, *et al.* Neuropsychological dysfunction following elective cardiac operation. I. Early assessment. *J Thorac Cardiovasc Surg* 1982;84:585–94

134. Legre R, Bardot J, Kevorkian B, *et al.* Evaluation of 106 free flaps. Analysis of the failures and the indications [in French]. *Ann Chir Plast Esthet* 1989;34:385–91

135. Ackermann R, Ebert T. Complications and late sequelae following radical cystectomy and supravesicle urinary diversion [in German]. *Urologe [A]* 1985;24:150–5

136. Hendry WF. Morbidity and mortality of radical cystectomy (1971–78 and 1978–85). *J R Soc Med* 1986;79:395–400

137. Jivegard L, Bergqvist D, Holm J, *et al.* Preoperative assessment of the risk for cardiac death following thrombo embolectomy for acute lower limb ischaemia. *Eur J Vasc Surg* 1992;6:83–8

138. Kepiantalo MJ, Haajanen J, Lindfors O, *et al.* Predictive value of preoperative segmental blood pressure measurements in below-knee amputations. *Acta Chir Scand* 1982;148:581–4

139. Kortmann H, Becker HM. Abdominal aortic aneurysms: diagnostic and surgical problems on advanced age [in German]. *Z Gerontol* 1985; 18:44–7

140. Schepens MA, Defauw JJ, Hamerlijnck PP, *et al*. Risk assessment of acute renal failure after thoracoabdominal aortic aneurysm surgery. *Ann Surg* 1994;219:400–7

141. Campbell WB, Ballard PK, Goodman DA. Intensive care after abdominal aortic surgery. *Eur J Vasc Surg* 1991;5:665–8

142. Bjerkelund CE, Smith-Erichsen N, Solheim K. Abdominal aortic reconstruction. Prognostic importance of coexistent diseases. *Acta Chir Scand* 1986;152:111–15

143. Rue LW 3rd, Cioffi WG, Mason AD, *et al*. Improved survival of burned patients with inhalation injury. *Arch Surg* 1993;128:772–8

144. Dean E, Ross J. Discordance between cardiopulmonary physiology and physical therapy. Toward a rational basis for practice. *Chest* 1992; 101:1694–8

145. Allman RM, Laprade CA, Noel LB, *et al*. Pressure sores among hospitalized patients. *Ann Intern Med* 1986;105:337–42

146. Allman RM, Walker JM, Hart MK, *et al*. Air-fluidized beds or conventional therapy for pressure sores: a randomized trial. *Ann Intern Med* 1987;107:641–8

147. Fink MP, Helsmoortel CM, Stein KL, *et al*. The efficacy of an oscillating bed in the prevention of lower respiratory tract infection in critically ill victims of blunt trauma: a prospective study. *Chest* 1990;97: 132–7

148. Cerrato D, Ariano C, Fiacchino F. Deep vein thrombosis and low-dose heparin prophylaxis in neurosurgical patients. *J Neurosurg* 1978;49: 378–81

149. Russell JC. Prophylaxis of postoperative deep vein thrombosis and pulmonary embolism. *Surg Gynecol Obstet* 1983;157:89–104

150. Oster G, Tuden RL, Colditz GA. Prevention of venous thromboembolism after general surgery. Cost-effectiveness analysis of alternative approaches to prophylaxis. *Am J Med* 1987;82:889–99

151. Stovsky B, Rudy E, Dragonette P. Comparison of two types of communication methods used after cardiac surgery with patients with endotracheal tubes. *Heart Lung* 1988;17:281–9

152. Knaus WA, Draper EA, Wagner DP, *et al*. Prognosis in acute organ-system failure. *Ann Surg* 1985;202:685–93

153. Crump JM, Duncan DA, Wears R. Analysis of multiple organ system failure in trauma and nontrauma patients. *Am Surg* 1988;54: 702–8

154. Darling GE, Duff JH, Mustard RA, *et al*. Multiorgan failure in critically ill patients. *Can J Surg* 1988;31:172–6
155. Manship L, McMillin RD, Brown JJ. The influence of sepsis and multisystem and organ failure on mortality in the surgical intensive care unit. *Am Surg* 1984;50:94–101
156. Tran DD, Van Onselen EB, Wensink AJ, *et al*. Factors related to multiple organ system failure and mortality in a surgical intensive care unit. *Nephrol, Dial, Transplant* 1994;4:172–8
157. Jennett B, Bond M. Assessment of outcome after severe brain damage: a practical scale. *Lancet* 1975;1:480–5
158. Cullen DJ, Civetta JM, Briggs BA, *et al*. Therapeutic intervention scoring system: a method for quantitative comparison of patient care. *Crit Care Med* 1974;2:57–60
159. Keene AR, Cullen DJ. Therapeutic intervention scoring system: update 1983. *Crit Care Med* 1983;11:1–3
160. Knaus WA, Zimmerman JE, Wagner DP, *et al*. APACHE – acute physiology and chronic health evaluation: a physiologically based classification system. *Crit Care Med* 1981;9:591–7
161. Brannen AL II, Godfrey LJ, Goetter WE. Prediction of outcome from critical illness: a comparison of clinical judgement with a prediction rule. *Arch Intern Med* 1989;149:1083–6
162. Escarce JJ, Kelley MA. Admission source to the medical intensive care unit predicts hospital death independent of APACHE II score. *J Am Med Assoc* 1990;264:2389–94
163. Knaus WA, Wagner DP, Draper EA, *et al*. The APACHE III prognostic system risk prediction of hospital mortality for critically ill hospitalized adults. *Chest* 1991;100:1619–36
164. Barie PS, Hydo LJ, Fischer E. Comparison of APACHE II and III scoring systems for mortality prediction in critical surgical illness. *Arch Surg* 1995;130:77–82
165. Le Gall JR, Phillippe L, Alperovitch A, *et al*. A simplified acute physiology score for ICU patients. *Crit Care Med* 1984;12:975–7
166. Lemeshow S, Teres D, Pastides H, *et al*. A method for predicting survival and mortality of ICU patients using objectively derived weights. *Crit Care Med* 1985;13:519–25
167. Dixon WJ, chief ed. *BMDP Statistical Software*, BMDP7M, Berkeley: University of California Press, 1981:519–37
168. Dixon WJ, chief ed. *BMDP Statistical Software*, BMDPLR, Berkeley: University of California Press, 1981:330–44
169. Lemeshow S, Teres D, Avrunin JS, *et al*. Refining intensive care unit outcome prediction by using changing probabilities of mortality. *Crit Care Med* 1988;16:470–7

170. Lemeshow S, Teres D, Avrunin JS, *et al*. Predicting the outcome of intensive care unit patients. *J Am Stat Assoc* 1988;83:348–56

171. Lemeshow S, Teres D, Kler J, *et al*. Mortality probability models (MPM II) based on an international cohort of intensive care unit patients. *J Am Med Assoc* 1993;270:2478–86

172. Le Gall JR, Lemeshow S, Saulnier F. A new simplified acute physiology score (SAPS II) based on a European/North American multicenter study. *J Am Med Assoc* 1993;270:2957–63

173. Lemeshow S, Hosmer DW Jr. A review of goodness of fit statistics for use in the development of logistic regression models. *Am J Epidemiol* 1982;115:92–106

174. Hanley JA, McNeil BJ. The meaning and use of the area under a receiver operating characteristic (ROC) curve. *Radiology* 1982;143: 29–36

175. Lemeshow S, Jean-Roger LG. Modeling the severity of illness of ICU patients: a systems update. *J Am Med Assoc* 1994;272:1049–55

176. Perkins HS, Jonsen AR, Epstein WV. Providers as predictors: using outcome predictions in intensive care. *Crit Care Med* 1986;14:105–10

177. Christensen C, Cottrell JJ, Murakami J, *et al*. Forecasting survival in the medical intensive care unit: a comparison of clinical prognoses with formal estimates. *Meth Inf Med* 1993;32:302–8

178. Miranda AF, Miranda S. Quality of life and long-term survival after intensive care discharge. *Med J Malaysia* 1991;46:66–71

179. Zimmerman JE, Knaus WA, Judson JA, *et al*. Patient selection for intensive care: a comparison of New Zealand and United States hospitals. *Crit Care Med* 1988;16:318–26

180. Ridley S, Plenderleith L. Survival after intensive care. Comparison with a matched normal population as an indicator of effectiveness. *Anaesthesia* 1994;49:933–5

181. Wesselink RM, van Staden RF, Leusink JA. Results of long-term intensive care in 223 patients [in Dutch]. *Nedelands Tijdschr Geneeskde* 1994;138:2247–51

3
Outcome of acute traumatic injury

Acute traumatic injury is a pervasive problem in modern Western society, predominantly a disease of the young (1–37 years) but with disability affecting all age groups. Nationally in the USA, the annual mortality rate for trauma is 140 000 persons with an additional 80 000 persons left with neurological disability[1]. This morbidity and mortality results in an estimated four million years of future working-life lost, twice that for ischemic heart disease or malignancy[1]. Predictors and correlates of outcome in the acutely injured trauma patient include mechanism (blunt or penetrating) and severity, as well as premorbid condition.

PREHOSPITAL CARE

The benefits of prehospital emergency medical service care have been debated. Controversy centers around the utility of aggressive intervention at the scene of injury relative to rapid transport to a facility for definitive care. Prospective evaluation by Potter and colleagues[2] of prehospital advanced life-support in 472 patients or basic life-support in 589 patients, which was associated with a field time of 17 min vs. 13 min, respectively, showed equivalent lengths of hospital stay and did not result in a difference of survival rates. However, a prospective cohort analysis of prehospital health-care resources by Schwartz and co-workers[3], comparing aeromedical transport of 673 patients from the accident scene with interhospital transport of 204 patients, demonstrated a decrease in hospital stay (from 18 to 12 days) and subsequent charges (from $US 16 734 to $US 8781) in the direct-from-scene transport group compared to ground transport. Evaluation of 387 patients requiring aeromedical transport found improved outcome, comparing the German system which utilized trauma surgeons and the American system relying on paramedics and nurses as flight personnel in populations controlled for injury severity[4].

TRAUMA SYSTEMS

Organized trauma systems with regulated prehospital care, aeromedical transport, triage, trauma center designation, quality assurance, specialty care, research, rehabilitation, public education and disaster planning have improved the outcome in acute traumatic injury[5].

The American College of Surgeons' standards for trauma centers issued in 1987 suggested that: level I centers should be staffed by in-house trauma surgery and anesthesiology physicians allowing them to treat 600–1000 patients annually; level II centers should be staffed by trauma surgery physicians on patient arrival and by anesthesiology physicians at or shortly after patient arrival, treating 350–600 patients annually; and level III centers, evaluating fewer than 350 trauma patients annually, should address nursing staff, facility, quality assurance and educational issues[5,6].

Recommendations from *Resources for optimal care of the injured patient* (1993) suggest that 800–1000 injured patients per million population require trauma center care, and general surgeons who manage 50 emergency trauma patients per year have adequate experience to participate in comprehensive trauma care[7]. The current system describes level I designation as a regional resource trauma center, usually a tertiary care referral institution, with most being university-based teaching hospitals. Clinical capabilities should emphasize subspecialty care, including cardiac surgery, hand surgery, microvascular (replantation) surgery, infectious disease, pediatric surgery and be complimented by the in-house capability of the general surgeon, while facilities/resources include cardiopulmonary bypass, operating microscope, acute hemodialysis, nuclear scanning and neuroradiology capability[7].

Level II facilities are expected to provide initial definitive trauma care, usually in a community setting and most commonly encountered, managing the majority of trauma patients. Level III facilities provide appropriate emergency intervention and stabilization using an on-call surgeon, and transfer to a level I/II facility when necessary. A new category, level IV, has been described to include clinic or aid-station facilities in remote, rural areas, which require treatment, stabilization and transfer protocols[7]. Thus, the most recent trauma care classification system emphasizes optimal use of the available resources to care for those suffering from accident or injury.

A historical comparison of 1108 patients in a major university hospital with a newly established trauma system showed a significant decrease in mortality (from 25 to 6%), an improvement in outcome for sepsis (from 29 to 15%) and a two-fold reduction in preventable complications[8]. Studies by Clemmer and colleagues[9] and Smith and associates[10], comparing designated trauma centers with community hospitals, showed a significant reduction in mortality as well as a decrease in morbidity in those hospitalized in the trauma centers. Mullins and co-workers[11] performed a retrospective cohort analysis of 70 350 hospitalized trauma patients in an urban multicenter trauma system, compared to historic controls. There was a significant decline in death rate, even with an increased injury severity score (>16) in those evaluated.

However, community hospitals that evaluate a moderate number of trauma patients (>200 patients) annually demonstrate equivalent mortality rates in matched-patient populations, suggested by a study of 752 blunt trauma cases by Waddell and colleagues[12]. Thus, one determinant of outcome may be the competence of the institution, based on the number of trauma patients treated annually (level I, > 600 patients; level II, >200–600 patients; and level III, < 200 patients). Likewise, comparison of rural programs yields similar findings of acceptable outcome for both geographically isolated high-volume level I or lower-volume level III centers[13,14]. Mechanism of injury as well as the effectiveness of trauma care may be an important determinant of survival. The survival rate for penetrating trauma was less than that for blunt trauma (20% vs. 29%) in Shackford and associates' evaluation[15] of 3394 patients with significant injury, where 283 (8.3%) had a trauma score of <8.

Medicolegal aspects of trauma practice may suggest a difference in care rendered at level I, compared to level II/III facilities. Analysis of the latter group demonstrates a two-fold increase in lawsuit incidence, as well as a 30% increase in cases resulting in litigation, in Weiland and colleagues' evaluation[16] of 191 trauma patients. The incidence of lawsuits was highest with the following types of conditions: fracture (14%), head or thoracic abdominal injury (8%), amputation (6%), cervical fracture (5%) and obstetric (4%) trauma cases. Cervical fracture ($US 3.5 million) and head injury ($US 2.5 million) were the most costly errors, with respect to monetary judgement per incident, in this sample[16].

The costs of trauma care related to personnel requirements have also been examined. The presence of an in-house trauma surgeon has been evaluated, and there was no difference in overall outcome (96% vs. 97%) or outcome in those with severe thoracoabdominal (76% vs. 81%) injury requiring operative intervention, comparing day and night shift arrival times in a sample of 3689 patients managed in a level II community setting[17]. Similarly, the relatively low incidence of surgical intervention required, which was 86 (13%) in a sample of 659 major trauma patients, and an equivalent response time (100 min) until surgery was commenced questioned the need for in-house operating room staff[18]. This study by Barone and co-workers[18] suggested equivalent times until surgery as well as similar mortality rates, comparing in-house with on-call operating room staff, realizing a cost saving of $US 145 000 annually.

PREDICTORS

Patients with pre-existing medical conditions had an increased mortality risk, based on logistic regression analysis, reported as a relative risk ratio of 4.5 for cirrhosis, 3.2 for coagulopathy, 1.8 for ischemic heart disease or chronic obstructive lung disease and 1.2 for diabetes, from Morris and colleagues' analysis of 3074 trauma patients[19].

Retrospective analysis by Morris and colleagues[20] of a 199 737 patient database found injury severity to be the most important determinant of survival, followed by age and pre-existing illness as described in their previous work. The presence of male gender and being of middle age (40–60 years) were previously underappreciated mortality correlates[20]. Although pre-existing organ system dysfunction, such as hepatic, cardiovascular, respiratory or renal involvement, or diabetes has a profound effect on patient outcome after controlling for age, mechanism and severity of injury, the relatively low incidence (5%) in some populations may not affect institutional outcome[21].

Age is an important factor in predicting outcome. Pediatric patients, on the whole, do better than adults, with a mortality rate of 6% (20 of 335)[22]. This approximate rate, however, increased four-fold (30 of 128) in tertiary pediatric care centers in Pollack and associates' multicenter evaluation[22]. Mortality rates adjusted for physiological profiles found an unexpected number of deaths in tertiary care centers, based on the severity of illness, while actual deaths (20 vs. 14) were greater than predicted in non-tertiary centers[22]. This finding is explained by an increase in the severity of illness, which warranted transfer to a tertiary care referral center, resulting in selection bias.

AGE

Nakayama and colleagues[23] analyzed a group of 4615 pediatric (<15 years) patients, comparing patients with the arbitrary age classifications 0–4, 5–9 and 10–14 years, to suggest that unadjusted mortality rates are decreased in older patients perhaps owing to developmental changes. However, after controlling for injury severity, there was no age-dependent mortality difference. Nevertheless, age criteria are still used in the determination of severity in pediatric injury scales such as the pediatric trauma score, where age is inversely correlated with severity[24].

The issue arises of the advisability of pediatric trauma care in the adult emergency setting. Knudson and co-workers[25] reviewed the cases of 353 injured children, demonstrating an unexpected mortality rate of only 6%, and favorable survival statistics with Z-scores ranging from +0.32 for toddlers (<2 years) to +3.98 for teenage children (14–17 years), compared to major trauma outcome study (MTOS) reference data[26]. Bensard and associates[27] also suggest that pediatric trauma patients may be triaged to the nearest regional trauma center, independent of adult or pediatric designation, based on their evaluation of 410 children (<15 years) and 188 young adults (16–18 years), comparing favorably in terms of survival (98.0% vs. 97.7%) estimated by therapeutic revised injury severity scale methodology, while the Z-statistic revealed no difference in outcome, compared to MTOS normals[26,27].

Geriatric trauma victims may not do as well as younger patients in the trauma setting, because of pre-existing health conditions and limited physiological reserve. There was no difference in mortality rate (8.6% vs. 6.0%) between geriatric (>65 years) and younger (<64 years) trauma patients during the initial period of care in Smith and colleagues' evaluation[28] of 63 patients. Mortality in geriatric patients was found to occur with less severe injury, according to the injury severity score, and increased progressively if patient complications occurred during the recovery phase[28].

Geriatric trauma victims with moderate injury severity, indicated by a mean score of >23, have poor outcomes, in the presence of concurrent craniocerebral trauma designated by a decreased Glasgow coma score (<7)[28]. Subsequent complications of shock, head injury or sepsis were found in a significant proportion (16%) of elderly patients[29]. Although the mortality rate was high (45%), those patients who were discharged returned to normal (17%) or independent (67%) living conditions in a significant proportion of cases in van Aalst and colleagues' analysis[29] of 98 geriatric trauma patients. Outcome in DeMaria and co-workers' study[30] of 68 geriatric patients was improved if they were analyzed later (>3 months) in the recovery phase, with improvement noted in recovery to independent living standards (from 33 to 56%), while the requirements decreased for dependent living (from 37 to 24%) conditions and nursing home placement (from 30 to 6%). The costs for intensive care unit (ICU) care in general and specifically for the geriatric patient population have been examined. Finelli and associates[31] compared 180 elderly (>65 years) major trauma patients with 3918 younger (<65 years) patients, demonstrating an increase in mortality between age 45 (10%) and 55 years (15%) with further worsening (20%) by age 75 years. The elderly had a two-fold increase in median length of stay (from 7 to 14 days), with increased infectious (4.6/100 vs. 0.7/100) and pulmonary (14/100 vs. 6.1/100) complications, and costs calculated using diagnostic-related groups (DRG) criteria grossly underestimated with a mean loss of $US 2177 per patient[31]. Grenrot and colleagues[32] evaluated the intensive care stay of 143 elderly patients (>70 years), and suggested that ICU cost per patient per year saved was not much higher for those with higher mortality rates or longer ICU stays, compared to the less severely ill patient groups[32].

Head injury may also influence outcome. Length of coma reflecting severity of brain damage was a better predictor of adverse outcome than other medical conditions and variables including age in Wilson and co-workers' study[33] of 115 head injury patients. Although age may contribute to improved overall outcome, young patients (15–44 years) may also have a higher rate of late behavioral and emotional sequelae based on Thomsen's evaluation of 40 trauma cases[34].

IMMUNE RESPONSE

Trauma is a significant activator of the immune system, initiating a complex cascade of humoral and cell-mediated inflammatory responses. Non-specific monitors of immune function include serum protein levels. Post-traumatic sepsis was associated with decreased levels of prealbumin, transferrin, fibronectin and antithrombin III ($p < 0.01$) in Rubli and associates' comparison[35] of 33 septic with 65 non-septic control trauma patients. Transferrin was found to be the most sensitive indicator, while antithrombin III was the most specific inflammatory mediator outcome marker, correlating inversely with survival[35].

Survey data from Christou and Tellado's evaluation[36] of 500 trauma–surgical ICU patients demonstrated abnormalities in leukocyte adherence and chemotaxis, while cell-mediated immunity, age and albumin levels were not correlated with poor outcome. However, the presence of a delayed hypersensitivity response to cutaneous testing was predictive of survival (77% vs. 23%) in the trauma population, in the 35-patient sample of Wolmann and Kress[37]. Similarly, a positive phytohemagglutinin response was associated with a two-fold decrease in mortality rate in 68 trauma patients, compared to those who were anergic (from 38 to 15%), in Visser and colleagues' study[38] of 275 critically ill surgical patients.

Newer diagnostic modalities involve monitoring of lymphocyte subsets or inflammatory mediator levels. Cell-mediated immunity has been related to sepsis in Kabisch and co-workers' study[39] of septic trauma patients who exhibited a decrease in cluster of differentiation cell types 2, 8 and 20 ($p < 0.01$), associated with a 67% (4 of 6) mortality rate, examining the progression of the preseptic (days 1–3), sepsis-development (days 3–6) and septic-disease (days 4–10) phases of illness[39]. Last, the presence of phospholipase A_2-activating protein, a marker of tissue damage, measured in urine (>12 nmol/l) by enzyme-linked immunosorbent assay (ELISA) was associated with poor outcome (i.e. death or a persistent vegetative state) in Fiennes and associates' analysis[40] of nine polytrauma patients.

CARDIAC INJURY

Patients with myocardial contusion or primary cardiac injury, as a result of blunt chest trauma, diagnosed by electrocardiographic and enzymatic standards, had a four-fold increase in mortality (27% vs. 6%) in Sturaitis and colleagues' evaluation[41] of 79 injured patients. Myocardial injury was manifested in this sample as right-sided heart dysfunction with a significant decrease in right-heart ejection fraction (from 47 ± 8 to $34 \pm 10\%$) ($p < 0.05$)[41]. Rady and co-workers' evaluation[42] of hemodynamic and oxygen transport patterns in 24 patients with initial cardiac dysfunction secondary to significant thoracic trauma, as denoted by decreased left-ventricular stroke work index, demonstrated worsening of cardiopulmonary variables, compared to those with relatively normal cardiac function. The abnormalities included decreases in stroke volume index, cardiac index (5.3 l/min/m^2 vs. 3.2 l/min/m^2), oxygen delivery (852 ml/min/m^2 vs. 469 ml/min/m^2) and mixed venous oxygen saturation (82% vs. 73%), and an increase in oxygen extraction index (19% vs. 29%) ($p < 0.001$). Mortality was increased six-fold (13% vs. 78%) in those patients with secondary cardiac dysfunction after chest injury in this observational study[42]. Thus, cardiac dysfunction occurring in patients secondary to significant traumatic injury may worsen overall outcome.

Geriatric blunt-trauma patients may benefit from early invasive hemodynamic monitoring to assist in diagnosis and management of occult cardiac dysfunction. Scalea and colleagues[43] reported that patients with severe myocardial dysfunction associated with cardiac output of <3.5 l/min and mixed venous oxygen saturation of < 50% suffered from 100% mortality in eight of 15 patients in the diagnostic phase. Survival improved to 53% (seven of 13) if early instrumentation (< 2.2 h) and therapeutic intervention were instituted, increasing cardiac output to at least 6.3 l/min[43].

PULMONARY INJURY

Markers for pulmonary injury include the presence of three or more rib fractures, which was associated with increased mortality (4%), injury severity score and length of intensive care and hospital stays ($p < 0.001$), in Lee and co-workers' retrospective analysis of 3282 blunt-trauma patients. The relative risks for associated injuries were 15.1 for hemothorax or pneumothorax, 6.5 for splenic rupture and 2.3 for hepatic laceration[44].

Mechanical ventilation after trauma, especially pulmonary contusion, is often complicated by infection, either tracheobronchitis (19%) or pneumonia (17%), as noted in Fussle and associates' study[45] of 190 patients. This sample suggests that 50% of the infectious complications of trauma are caused by *Pseudomonas aeruginosa, Staphylococcus aureus* or *Streptococcus* species[45]. Newer emerging pathogens include *Acinetobacter anitratus, Enterobacter cloacae, E. aerogenes* and *Enterococcus faecium* in the trauma as well as the general intensive care population.

RENAL FAILURE

The onset of acute renal failure during the intensive care course may be predicted by preoperative abnormal creatinine level or advanced age, and may increase the length of hospital stay, morbidity and mortality, as shown in Corwin and colleagues' sample[46] of 572 cardiac surgery patients. Factors predisposing to acute renal failure, ultimately requiring hemodialysis, included sepsis (100%), hypotension (43%) and nephrotoxic drugs or dye in 33% of 21 surgical ICU patients, in Mukau and Latimer's evaluation[47] of acute hemodialysis in the critically ill. In those with persistent creatinine clearance of < 40 ml/min, ICU mortality was 100%, compared to 80% in those with normal creatinine clearance[47]. Similarly, in the trauma or surgical ICU population of 100 consecutive patients reported by Wheeler and co-workers[48], survival may be worsened in those aged over 50 years and a serum creatinine level greater than 6.0 mg/dl.

GASTROINTESTINAL INJURY

Solid organ injuries, such as severe hepatic trauma, often predispose the patient to a prolonged hospital course; however, the length of stay (decreased from 40 to 20 days) and the complication rate may be minimized by ICU intervention, based on the work of Foco and associates[49]. A frequent complication of critical illness in the trauma population is acute acalculous cholecystitis. Patients are predisposed to this condition if they have a prolonged ICU stay (100%) or narcotic therapy (100%), or receive total parenteral nutrition in 93% of cases, as demonstrated in Cornwell and colleagues' observational study[50] of 14 patients. Ultrasound and computed tomography often revealed an increase in wall thickness (>4 mm), pericholecystic fluid, intramucosal gas and tissue sloughing. There was a 7% mortality rate in trauma patients in this sample with acalculous cholecystitis[50].

ORTHOPEDIC INJURY

Orthopedic injury is perhaps the most common finding in Wardrope and co-workers' study[51] of 1577 patients with blunt trauma, of which 695 (44%) were admitted, with a ten-fold greater predominance of bony injury (62%), compared to visceral (6%) trauma. Most admissions, 62% (421/678), were for an isolated orthopedic injury, with serious injury (injury severity score >15) found in only 7% (43/678)[51]. A tertiary survey performed in the ICU setting identified injuries predominantly of extremity (5%) and axial spine (1%) fractures, which were not identified in 9% of patients in the primary or secondary survey performed in the emergency department, as reported in Enderson and colleagues' study[52] of 399 trauma patients.

The presence of an isolated femoral neck fracture in the elderly may have a mortality rate as high as 59% (36 of 61), according to Wardrope and co-workers' major trauma outcome study of 695 patients[51]. Similarly, patients with open contaminated pelvic fracture may have a mortality rate as high as 50%, often due to complications such as pulmonary embolism or infection. However, Poole and associates' survey[53] of 236 pelvic fracture patients suggested that fracture variables including site, displacement, stability and vector of injury are correlated with severity of injury ($p < 0.01$), but not with outcome itself. The study analyzed a more representative patient population instead of the geriatric cohort and found a 7.6% overall mortality rate.

INFECTION

Risk factors for infection in the surgical ICU include nutritional status, the presence of diabetes mellitus or cancer, splenectomy, steroid use, decreased lymphocyte count and shock states ($p < 0.05$)[54]. Manship and colleagues' evaluation[54] of sepsis in 77 surgical ICU patients suggests that 50% of ICU mortality was due to multisystem organ failure, and 60% of these fatalities could be directly attributed to sepsis[54]. There was an associated decrease in multisystem organ failure in trauma (21%, 11 of 53), compared to non-trauma (72%, 66 of 91) patients,

148

possibly because of fewer premorbid medical conditions in trauma cases[54]. Multisystem organ disease most frequently involved the cardiovascular (85%), pulmonary (83%) and renal (78%) systems, often associated with precipitating factors of shock (65%), ischemic heart disease (49%) or gastrointestinal bleeding (48%)[54].

Sepsis frequently arises in the setting of positive blood (65%) or sputum (47%) cultures. These cultures are significant for Gram-negative rods (76%), often *Pseudomonas aeruginosa* or *Klebsiella pneumoniae*, Gram-positive cocci (58%), such as *Staphylococcus aureus* or *Enterococcus*, and fungal species (27%), resulting in a mortality rate of 59% in bacteremic states with accompanying systemic inflammatory response[54].

HEAD INJURY

Perhaps the most significant variable in predicting outcome from traumatic injury is the presence of concomitant head injury. Survey data from Levi and co-workers' 64-patient military injury model[55] indicated that cerebral concussion or diffuse axonal injury was found most commonly in 23% of patients, followed by hematoma or contusion in 17% and hemorrhage in 11%, with head injury[55]. This experience with closed head injuries in the military setting showed that aggressive surgical intervention attempted in over half of the cases resulted in decreased mortality (19%) and surprisingly good outcome in 69% of patients, with only minimal to moderate residual dysfunction, compared to similar injuries in civilians[55].

Clinical examination often yields useful information regarding the likelihood of patient recovery. Assessment of the triad of Glasgow coma score, deep tendon reflexes and pupillary reactivity obtained 24 h after injury may help accurately to predict head injury outcome in children[56]. Predictive variables in adults also include Glasgow coma score (recorded at 6 h), age, associated injury, mechanism of injury, blood pressure, spontaneous ventilation and computed tomography findings, according to Waxman and colleagues' survey[57] of 306 severe head injury patients.

The Glasgow coma score, on presentation to the emergency department measured after resuscitative effort, may impact on mortality, based on information from the traumatic coma data bank, enrolling 1030 consecutive severely (Glasgow coma score < 8) head-injured patients, where 76% of those with post-resuscitation Glasgow score of < 3 died, compared to 18% of those with scores of 6–8[58]. The Glasgow coma score is probably the most reliable and reproducible early predictor of outcome, with examination periods ranging from 0 to 24 h after resuscitative efforts[56–58].

The anatomical nature and location of head injury are also important. Lesions that are amenable to surgical intervention, such as epidural hematoma, are often associated with better survival than lesions amenable to medical management, such as diffuse axonal injury, based on Meier and co-workers' evaluation[59] of 733 head-injured patients. Post-traumatic coma, defined as a state of unconsciousness persisting for at least 2 weeks, occurred in only a very small percentage (0.6%) of 135 traumatic head injury patients studied by Bricolo and associates[60]. Post-traumatic coma has been associated with the presence of an extracranial injury or a diencephalic lesion, as well as decerebrate posturing on presentation ($p < 0.01$)[60].

The widespread availability of computed tomography has generated several novel neurological injury classification systems. Andrews and associates[61] evaluated the anatomical location of intracranial lesions in 45 patients with head injuries, discovering that the frontal lobes (40%) were most commonly involved, followed by temporoparietal (38%) and parieto-occipital (22%) regions. Herniation syndromes were associated with either location of lesion, temporal or temporoparietal, in 41% or size of fluid collections, with lesions greater than 30 ml demonstrating a 64% incidence of herniation, both resulting in worsened outcome[61].

The traumatic coma data bank was used to develop a more elaborate diagnosis and classification system for head injury, based on computed tomography scan[62]. Diffuse brain injury is graded on a four-point scale, with normal (grade I), abnormal brain with cistern normal (grade II), cistern abnormal (grade III) or midline shift (grade IV). The likelihood of good outcome decreases (from 27 to 3%) and mortality increases (from 10 to 56%) with increasing scores derived from the computed tomography grading scale[62]. Outcomes of head injury associated with a mass lesion were worse when associated with volume >25 ml, the need for surgical evacuation, inability to evacuate the lesion or brain stem injury, while diffuse injury was worsened in the presence of a 5-mm midline shift[62]. Overall, good outcomes occurred in only 0–5% of the 1030 head injury patients studied (presenting with Glasgow coma scores <8), and mortality rates were in a range of 39–67% in each separate prognostic category[62].

The use of neurosurgical intensive care may facilitate the diagnosis and therapy of primary and secondary brain injuries. Warme and colleagues' prospective evaluation[63] of 121 severe head injury patients with similar injury severities suggested a three-fold improvement in outcome of patients treated in a neurosurgical, compared to general surgery, ICU. The most severely affected subgroup, with Glasgow scores <4, may benefit significantly from therapy targeted at preventing secondary brain injury, by optimizing cerebral blood flow and oxygen delivery.

A distinctive feature of neurosurgical intensive care is monitoring and treatment of intracranial pressure (ICP), which has detrimental effects on cerebral blood flow. The incidence of ICP elevation on presentation after head injury was 82% for minor elevation (ICP >10 mmHg), 44% for moderate elevation (ICP > 20 mmHg) and 10% for severe elevation of intracranial pressure (ICP > 40 mmHg) in Miller and co-workers' study[64] of 1601 patients. Poor outcome was noted, with minor ICP elevation associated with two extremes: either diffuse axonal injury or a mass lesion, resulting in surgical intervention in half of the cases and a 30% mortality rate in head-injured patients[64].

Thus, neurological outcome is dependent on proper regulation of cerebral blood flow and subsequent oxygen delivery. Poor outcome may be associated with sustained ICP elevation (>20 mmHg), as well as systemic hypotension (systolic blood pressure < 80 mmHg) occurring in as many as 74% of head injury patients, cited from the 654 trauma coma data bank patients who underwent ICP monitoring[65]. However, the most significant correlate is the cerebral perfusion pressure (CPP) or the net perfusion gradient to the brain, measured as the difference between mean arterial pressure (MAP) and ICP, expressed simplistically as the equation CPP = MAP – ICP. Cerebral perfusion pressure varies directly with cerebral blood flow (CBF) and inversely to cerebral vascular resistance (CVR), expressed as the relationship CPP = CBF/CVR. The actual incidence of CPP reduction (< 60 mmHg) in Stocchetti and associates' group of 121 head-injured patients[66] was 16%, and was minimized by autoregulatory increases in MAP to counteract the ICP elevation, which was preserved in more than 77% of head-injured patients.

The presence of head injury has both immediate and delayed effects on survival after acute traumatic injury. The institution of established head injury management programs, utilizing aggressive therapy, including early computed tomography and surgical drainage of intracranial hematoma or hemorrhage, has resulted in decreased length of hospital stay with mortality rates decreased from 45 to 34% in Miller and associates' 3-year evaluation[67] of regional head-trauma centers. Mortality is linearly proportional to age in those patients with severe head injury. Mortality was estimated at 33% in those 15–25 years of age, compared to 81% in those over 55 years of age, in the traumatic coma data bank head injury sample[68].

Secondary brain injury may occur in the ICU setting, owing to cerebral swelling and subsequent oxygen supply and demand mismatch. Shackford and colleagues' retrospective analysis[69] of fatalities in significant trauma demonstrated a preponderance of central nervous system injury (48%) with two-thirds of patients manifesting signs of secondary brain injury at autopsy. Retrospective analysis of trauma fatalities suggests a preponderance of central nervous system injury in 49% of patients with primary brain injury in one-third and secondary insult in two-thirds, associated with a mortality rate as high as 35% in those requiring admission to a neurosurgical ICU[58,69]. Simplistic analysis of head injury morbidity in Crawford's evaluation[70] of 51 ICU patients suggested that complete or moderate recovery may be achieved in 10% and 25% of patients, respectively. Analysis of the traumatic coma data bank demonstrated a diverse range of outcomes from severe head trauma associated with a Glasgow coma score of < 8, ranging from good recovery in 7% to moderate disability in 18%, severe disability in 28%, persistent vegetative state in 14% and death in 33% of those evaluated[71].

A more valid prediction of patient outcome may be based upon analysis later in the recovery phase, at 1 year for adults and 5 years for children. Examination of neurological outcome at 1 year suggested good recovery in up to 13% of patients, moderate disability in at least 18%, severe disability in up to 31% and persistent vegetative state in at least 8%, while up to 30% did not survive (Table 1)[60,61,71,72].

Perhaps the most devastating condition for the patient and family is the persistent vegetative state, in which there is apparent wakefulness, but not cognitive awareness. Persistent vegetative state was found in 14% of patients (93 of 650) referred for analysis from the traumatic coma data bank and was associated with initial low Glasgow coma scores, abnormal pupillary findings or the onset of diabetes insipidus[72].

Table 1 Outcome associated with severe head injury. Data from references 60, 61, 71 and 72

	Incidence (%)	
	Range	*Cumulative*
Recovery		
Good	7–13	10
Disability		
Moderate	18–25	21
Severe	28–31	29
Persistent vegetative state	8–14	22
Mortality	3–30	16

During the recovery process it was found that, by 6 months, 41% of the patients regained consciousness, followed by 52% at 1 year and 68% 3 years after traumatic injury[72]. Long-term outcome analysis performed by Glinz and Ruckert[73], 5 years after traumatic injury, demonstrated that the presence of severe head injury adversely impacts upon the likelihood of successful rehabilitation, with full recovery found in 82% (59 of 72) without head injury, but only 45% (30 of 66) of those with significant head injury were fully reintegrated into society.

SPINAL CORD INJURY

Spinal cord injury is a particularly devastating form of neurological dysfunction. DeVivo and colleagues' study[74] of 5131 spinal cord injury patients admitted to regional spinal cord injury centers reported an overall mortality rate of 9% in those who survived the first 24 h, predominantly owing to pneumonia and unintentional suicide or injury.

Therapy by Bracken and co-workers[75] with methylprednisolone (30 mg/kg bolus and 5.4 mg/kg infusion for 23 h) administered within 8 h of traumatic spinal cord injury resulted in improvement in both sensory and motor assessment scores at 6 months post-injury. Geisler and associates[76] performed a prospective placebo-controlled, double-blinded trial of GM-1 ganglioside in 34 spinal cord injury patients, noting functional improvement measured as the Frankel score and motor improvement measured as the American Spinal Injury

Association score[77,78]. The former study emphasized a sensitive outcome scale, while the latter study focused on a specific recovery scale. Outcome analysis suggested a 4% case fatality rate during hospitalization for spinal cord injury, while 24% of those with thoracolumbar injury and 36% with cervical injury experienced later neurological recovery in Gerhart's study[79] of 358 spinal cord injury patients. Most (95%) patients were discharged home, with two-thirds rating their adjustment and quality of life as good or excellent[79]. Heinemann and colleagues' study[80] comparing the functional outcome of 185 patients who underwent specialized short-term spinal cord injury care, compared to general hospital care, reported improved functional gains demonstrated during long-term rehabilitation in the intervention group.

MULTISYSTEM ORGAN FAILURE

Organ system dysfunction may also be categorized and used to predict outcome. Knaus and co-workers[81] analyzed 5677 consecutive general surgery ICU admissions and found that failure of a single organ system persisting for at least 48 h resulted in up to 40% mortality, which increased to 60% with two systems, and up to 98% of patients not surviving an ICU stay if failure of three systems occurred. There is a progressive linear increase in mortality with increase in the number of organ systems involved, from a baseline of no systems (1% mortality) to seven systems (86% mortality) (Table 2)[81–83]. Similar analyses of 203

Table 2 Outcome associated with organ system failure in surgical patients. Data from references 81–83

	Mortality (%)	
Number of organ systems	*Absolute or range*	*Cumulative*
0	1	
1	13–40	26
2	34–60	47
3	45–98	73
4	83–93	88
5	68	
6	96	
7	86	

patients by Crump and associates[82] and 1136 trauma and non-trauma surgical patients by Darling and colleagues[83] suggested that another important consideration is the specific organ system involved. The pulmonary system was most commonly affected in surgical (78%) and trauma patients (83%) (Table 3)[82,83]. Persistent cardiovascular system involvement resulted in the most significant mortality, found in 79% of surgical patients and 100% of trauma patients[82,83].

Knaus and co-workers' comparison[81] of 481 trauma with non-trauma surgical patients suggests that the incidence of multisystem organ failure is increased two-fold in traumatic injury. However, there was a 50% reduction in the incidence of sepsis and subsequent mortality associated with multisystem organ failure in the trauma population[81,84].

SCORING SYSTEMS

Organized scoring systems may be classified into two categories: initial triage scales and final outcome scales. Triage assessment tools include the Glasgow coma scale (GCS), perhaps the most widely used reproducible grading scale; however, it was designed to be used with craniocerebral trauma[85]. The trauma score (TS) gleaned from analysis of a 2000-patient group combines neurological assessment with cardiopulmonary variables, including the respiratory rate and effort, systolic blood pressure, capillary refill and GCS score[86]. It is the second most common rating scale and is widely used successfully by pre-hospital personnel, nurses and physicians[86]. The revised trauma score (RTS) selected systolic blood pressure (SBP) and respiratory rate (RR) as the most significant cardiopulmonary variables, as well as increasing the relative importance of the neurological examination (GCS) (Table 4)[87]. The revised trauma score is the current triage standard, in which variables are grouped into a five-tier system with coded values of 0–4. This equation is expressed as $RTS = 0.9368GCS_c + 0.7326SBP_c + 0.2908RR_c$, with coefficient weights based on population data coded to a reference scale[87].

The pediatric trauma score (PTS) developed by Tepas and colleagues[24] rates six injury factors including patient size, airway integrity, SBP, central nervous system involvement, open wound injuries and skeletal injury into three categories (+2, +1, –1) with an overall score range of –6 to 12 (Table 5)[24]. There is a linear relationship between PTS

Table 3 Specific organ system involvement in trauma and surgical patients. Data from references 82 and 83

| | Trauma | | Surgical | | | |
| | | | Mortality (%) | | Incidence (%) | |
Organ system	Mortality (%)	Incidence (%)	Range	Cumulative	Range	Cumulative
Cardiovascular	100	9	70–89	79	11–84	47
Hematological	80	9	56–86	71	17–45	31
Renal	59	23	69–74	71	44–63	53
Gastrointestinal	50	8	39–72	55	22–27	24
Hepatic	50	11	64–65	64	21–50	35
Central nervous system	39	53	47–69	58	39–86	62
Pulmonary	33	83	50–63	56	74–83	78

Table 4 Triage scoring systems: adult, revised trauma score. Table adapted from reference 87

	Glasgow Coma Scale score				
Variable	13–15	9–12	6–8	4–5	3
Systolic blood pressure (mmHg)	>89	76–89	50–75	1–49	0
Respiratory rate (breaths/min)	10–29	>29	6–9	1–5	0
Coded value	4	3	2	1	0

Table 5 Triage scoring systems: pediatric, pediatric trauma score. Table adapted from reference 24

	Category		
Variable	+2	+1	−1
Size (kg)	≥ 20	10–20	< 10
Airway	normal	maintainable	unmaintainable
Systolic blood pressure (mmHg)	≥ 90	90–50	< 50
Central nervous system	awake	loss of consciousness	coma/ decerebrate
Open wound	none	minor	major/ penetrating
Skeletal	none	closed fracture	open/multiple fractures

and injury severity scale (ISS) ($p < 0.001$) and similar regression co-efficients (−3.50, −3.77) when the 110-patient study group is compared to the 120-patient national pediatric trauma registry baseline[24]. However, Kaufmann and associates' comparison[88] found no advantage of substituting pediatric for adult trauma score, noting both a decrease in triage accuracy (from 79 to 68%) and the standard difficulties of implementing a new classification system.

The circulation respiration abdomen motor and speech scale (CRAMS) is a highly reproducible prehospital triage tool, which was obtained from analysis of 500 patients[89]. Major trauma is defined as CRAMS score of <8, while minor trauma is defined as CRAMS score of >9, although this scale has largely been replaced by the GCS and TS in trauma practice today[89]. The abbreviated injury scale (AIS) is a descriptive scale of motor vehicle-induced tissue damage classified into five body regions and nine levels of severity[90]. The most severe injury classification categories (6–9), all of which result in mortality, were eliminated in favor of a revised five-stage severity scale (1–5)[91]. The revised AIS score combines these moribund categories into a single designation (6), suggesting no further computation is necessary[92]. The AIS-85 revision modified the pre-existing scale into six body regions and five severity grades, to interpret more accurately those suffering from penetrating trauma[93,94]. The AIS-EM modification incorporated epidemiological classification techniques based on medical record and coding analysis, resulting in a significant decrease (from 68 to 15%) in unclassified injuries, as well as an increase in identification of head injury (from 16 to 37%)[95]. The AIS and ISS are more reliable when used by nurses and physicians than by emergency medical technicians or non-clinical technicians, and when used for blunt rather than penetrating trauma[96]. The ISS obtained from analysis of 2128 blunt trauma patients uses the sum of the squares of the three most severely injured regions, correcting for the quadratic rather than linear nature of the AIS progression, allowing for worsened outcome in those with multiple injuries[90]. The ISS allows retrospective comparison of trauma ICU patients, and is the standard for anatomical injury rating scales.

Thus, sensitivity, or the probability that the condition is present if the test is positive, is indicated by the likelihood of triage criteria activation of the trauma team when ISS is >15. Specificity, or the probability that the condition is absent if the test is negative, is indicated by the absence of triage criteria activation when ISS is <15. If the sensitivity of the screening tool decreases then the rate of undertriage increases, while if the specificity decreases then the rate of overtriage increases (Table 6)[85–91].

The outcome assessment scales include the comprehensive injury scale (CIS), which is the AIS companion functional outcome prediction system rating five factors (energy dissipation, threat to life, permanent impairment, treatment period or incidence) on a 1–5 scale with a range of outcome from 5 to 75, worsening with injury severity[97].

The Glasgow outcome scale (GOS) provides a descriptive analysis of functional outcome in patients with traumatic injury[98]. The therapeutic intervention scoring system (TISS) grades the utility of 57 ICU interventions and evaluates the efficacy of personnel, equipment, resource utilization and staffing[99]. The TISS 1983 update increased the analysis

Table 6 Triage scoring systems. Data from references 85–91

Method	Variables	Scale	Range	Monitor	Accuracy (%)	Sensitivity (%)	Specificity (%)
						Prediction	
Glasgow coma scale (GCS)	motor	1–6	3–15	craniocerebral trauma			
	verbal	1–5					
	eye opening	1–4					
Trauma score	respiratory rate	1–4	2–16	cardiopulmonary variables	95	80	70
	respiratory effort	0–1					
	systemic blood pressure	0–4					
	capillary repair	0–2					
	Glasgow coma scale	1–5					
Revised trauma score	blood pressure	0–4	0–12	triage (integer)	79–97	97	
	respiratory rate	0–4	0–8	outcome (non-integer)			
	Glasgow coma scale	0–4					
Pediatric trauma score	size, airway, SBP, CNS, open wound, skeletal trauma	+2,+1,–1	–6–12	pediatric survival	68		

Table 6 Continued over

Table 6 *Continued*

Method	*Variables*	*Scale*	*Range*	*Monitor*	Prediction		
					Accuracy (%)	*Sensitivity (%)*	*Specificity (%)*
Circulation respiration abdomen motor speech (CRAMS)	circulation respiration abdomen motor speech	0–2 0–2 0–2 0–2 0–2	0–10	prehospital triage		92	98
Abbreviated injury scale (AIS)	most severe AIS grade: general, head/neck, chest, abdominal, extremities/ pelvic girdle	0, no injury; 1, minor; 2, moderate; 3, severe (not life-threatening); 4, severe (life-threatening, survival probable); 5, critical (survival uncertain); 6, fatal (within 24 h + severity code 3); 7, fatal (within 24 h + severity code 4–5); 8, fatal (2 regions); 9, fatal (3 regions)	0–5	descriptive body region severity	non-linear correlation		

Table 6 Continued

160

Table 6 *Continued*

Method	Variables	Scale	Range	Monitor	Prediction		
					Accuracy (%)	Sensitivity (%)	Specificity (%)
Injury severity scale (ISS)	sum of squares of 3 AIS grades: $ISS = AIS_1^2 + AIS_2^2 + AIS_3^2$; external, head, neck, thorax, abdomen/pelvic contents, spine, extremities/bony pelvis	0–5: 1, minor; 2, moderate; 3, severe, not life-threatening; 4, severe, life-threatening; 5, critical, survival uncertain	0–75	retrospective group comparison	quadratic correlation, multisystem injury increased effect on mortality		

SBP, systolic blood pressure; CNS, central nervous system

to 76 ICU therapeutic maneuvers, graded on a 1–4 scale with only the maximal score for like interventions included[100]. Regression analysis using the $y = 0.5 + 1.03x$ relationship reveals a similar line of identity for both the 1974 and the 1983 scoring systems[99,100]. The therapeutic revised injury severity scale (TRISS) estimates the probability of survival evaluating age, anatomy or physiological variables[101].

The patient's age and premorbid condition, combined with illness variables, are the basis of the acute physiology and chronic health evaluation (APACHE) system. APACHE I evaluated 805 ICU admissions and classified health indicators and physiological variables to achieve an 81% accuracy[102]. APACHE II evaluated 5815 ICU admissions, and added an age criterion and decreased the significance of physiological variables to achieve 86% accuracy[103]. The current standard, APACHE III, based on 17 440 ICU patients, uses age, comorbid illness and physiological variables in a predictive equation model to achieve 88–95% classification accuracy[104]. However, the latter system is largely computer based and applicable to retrospective analysis of injury severity, rather than early triage of patients. The multiple logistic regression model uses nine disease indicators and physiological variables derived from a group of 755 patient admissions to achieve 87% accuracy in a simpler application model, but is validated in a smaller population sample[105] (Table 7)[98–105].

OUTCOME

The typical mortality rate after admission for critical illness to a general surgery ICU was 12%, compared to 20% in general-ward patients, from Zimmerman and colleagues' evaluation[106] of 5030 American and 1005 New Zealand ICU admissions. Kaukinen and co-workers' analysis[107] of the trauma population showed a comparable mortality rate of 23% in 228 ICU patients, which increased to 37% after 1 year in the severely injured, with the 1-year mortality rate of 58% highest in those with brain injury. Schiowitz's evaluation[108] of smaller trauma centers with an average of only 28 cases annually reports a mortality rate of 7% (6 of 85), with surprisingly little correlation to age or mechanism. Variables associated with greater mortality in Beeko and associates' 310 trauma-patient group[109] included age, need for craniotomy or thoracotomy, and neurological compromise measured as a decreased GCS or increased ICP on presentation.

Table 7 Outcome scoring systems. Data from references 98–105

Method	Variables	Scale	Range	Monitor	Prediction		
					Accuracy (%)	Sensitivity (%)	Specificity (%)
Comprehensive injury scale (CIS)	1, energy dissipation; 2, threat to life; 3, permanent impairment; 4, treatment period; 5, incidence	0–5	5–75	functional outcome			
Glasgow outcome scale (GOS)	1, death; 2, persistent vegetative state; 3, severe disability; 4, moderate disability; 5, good recovery	0–5	0–5	functional outcome			
Therapeutic intervention scoring system (TISS)	57 ICU interventions; 1, active transplant; 2, ICU personnel; 3, ICU technology; 4, standard code	1–4	0–70	resource staffing budget		96	95

Table 7 Continued over

Table 7 *Continued*

Method	*Variables*	*Scale*	*Range*	*Monitor*	*Accuracy (%)*	*Sensitivity (%)*	*Specificity (%)*
					Prediction		
Therapeutic revised injury severity scale (TRISS)	P_s = ISS + RTS + age: anatomical variables; physiological variables; age		0.0–1.0	survival		81	99
A severity characterization of trauma (ASCOT)	P_s: body region, 4 areas; RTS; age, 5 levels		0.0–1.0	survival		86	99
Acute physiology and chronic health evaluation (APACHE) system	I: 4 health indications, 34 physiological variables	0–4	0–50	survival	81	97	49
	II: age, general health, 12 physiological variables	0–4	0–71	survival	86	47	95
	III: age, comorbid conditions 20 physiological variables	0–24	0–299 0–23 0–252	predictive equation	88–95	13	99

Table 7 Continued

Table 7 *Continued*

Method	Variables	Scale	Range	Monitor	Prediction		
					Accuracy (%)	Sensitivity (%)	Specificity (%)
Multiple logistic regression (MLR) model	9 variables: age, systolic pressure, heart rate, organ failure, medical/ surgical, infection, CPR, elective/ emergency, level of consciousness			regression	87	50	96

ICU, intensive care unit; P_s, probability of survival; ISS, injury severity scale; RTS, revised trauma score; PS, probability of survival; CPR, cardiopulmonary resuscitation

OUTCOME PREDICTION

The major trauma outcome study (MTOS) analyzed information on 80 544 patients from 139 hospitals gathered from 1982 to 1989 by Champion and colleagues[26]. The overall mortality rate was 9.0% owing to blunt (34.7%) or penetrating (21.0%) trauma, with the presence of head injury strongly influencing mortality ranging from 5.0% (AIS < 3) to 40% (AIS > 4)[26]. The TRISS methodology estimates the survival probability P_s as the logistic function $P_s = 1/(1 + e^{-b})$ where e is the base of the natural logarithm (2.718 282) and $b = b_0 + b_1$ (TS or RTS) $+ b_2$(ISS) $+ b_3$(age)[26,101]. The normal regression weights were calculated from an initial 23 177-patient group, while age is equivalent to 0 if <54 years and age equals 1 if >55 years of age (Figure 1 and Table 8)[26].

The TRISS methodology has evolved from the use of the TS, which was essentially a triage instrument adapted to predict survival ranging from 0% (TS 1) to 99% (TS 16), to the RTS used currently. The RTS was modified after analysis of the MTOS initial 23 177-patient database, suggesting the significance of SBP, RR and GCS, and their importance expressed as whole numbers ranging from 0 to 4, modified by weighting factors, ranking their importance as GCS (0.936 81), SBP (0.7326) and RR (0.2908)[101]. Similarly, the ISS variable uses the 1985 AIS revision modified from the original Committee on Medical Aspects of Automotive Safety document 1971–72[90,97]. However, clinical validation of the original model suggested the TS/RTS variable required significant modification compared to ISS or age criteria, which were largely unchanged.

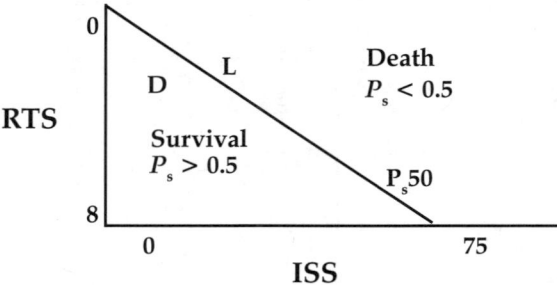

Figure 1 Therapeutic revised injury severity scale (TRISS) analysis. RTS, revised trauma score; ISS, injury severity scale; P_s, probability of survival

Table 8 Survival statistics: probability of survival of individual. Data from references 26, 91, 94, 101, 110, 111 and 113

	Trauma	
Reference values	*Blunt*	*Penetrating*
TRISS: 1983 (AIS-80)		
b_0 constant	−1.6465	−0.8068
b_1 TS	0.5175	0.5442
b_2 ISS	−0.0739	−0.1159
b_3 age	−1.9261	−2.4782
MTOS: 1990 (AIS-85)		
b_0 constant	−1.2470	−0.6029
b_1 RTS	0.9544	1.1430
b_2 ISS	−0.0768	−0.1516
b_3 age	−1.9052	−2.6676
MTOS: 1995 (AIS-90)		
b_0 constant	−0.4999	−2.5355
b_1 RTS	0.8085	0.9934
b_2 ISS	−0.0835	−0.0651
b_3 age	−1.7430	−1.1360

TRISS analysis
See Figure 1. D is unexpected death, L is unexpected survivor

Probability of survival

$$P_s = \frac{1}{1 + e^{-b}}$$

where   e = 2.718 282,   age = 0   (<54   years)   or   1   (≥ 55   years), $b = b_0 + b_1(\text{RTS}) + b_2(\text{ISS}) + b_3(\text{age})$

Injury severity
   $\text{RTS} = 0.9368 \ (\text{GCS}_c) + 0.7326 \ (\text{SBP}_c) + 0.2908 \ (\text{RR}_c)$
   $\text{ISS} = \text{AIS}_1^2 + \text{AIS}_2^2 + \text{AIS}_3^2$

Table 8 Continued over

Table 8 *Continued*

	Trauma	
Reference values	*Blunt*	*Penetrating*

Example

A 63-year-old male presents with fall from height with GCS (8), SBP (70 mmHg) and RR = 40. Injuries include a basilar skull fracture (AIS 3), bilateral hemothorax (AIS 4) and minor L1 compression fracture (AIS 2). Using GCS 8, GCS_c = 2; SBP 70, SBP_c = 2; RR 40, RR_c = 3:

$$RTS = 0.9368(2) + 0.7326(2) + 0.2908(3)$$
$$= 1.8736 + 1.4652 + 0.8724$$
$$= 4.2112$$

$$ISS = 3^2 + 4^2 + 2^2$$
$$= 29$$

$$b = -1.2470 + [0.9544(4.2112)] + [-0.0768(29)] + [-1.9052(1)]$$
$$= (-1.2470) + (4.0192) + (-2.272) + (-1.9052)$$
$$= -1.3602$$

$$P_s = \frac{1}{1 + 2.718\ 282^{-1.3602}}$$
$$= 0.2042$$

Probability of survival is 20.4%

TRISS, therapeutic revised injury severity scale; MTOS, major trauma outcome study; AIS, abbreviated injury scale; TS, trauma score; ISS, injury severity scale; RTS, revised trauma score; GCS, Glasgow coma score; SBP, systolic blood pressure; RR, respiratory rate

Patient outcome was presented using two mortality prediction models[26]. Preliminary outcome-based evaluation derives a 50% probability of survival (S50) regression line with ISS (*x* axis) plotted against TS (*y* axis)[110]. Thus, combinations of TS/ISS falling below the S50 isobar have a >50% survival probability, while those found above this line have a <50% survival probability. This analytical method serves a quality assurance function where qualitative predictions focus on unexpected deaths rather than survivors[110].

Definitive outcome-based evaluation allows comparison of two patient groups: the study and baseline populations expressed as the Z-statistic[7,26]. The Z-statistic is equivalent to (A – E)/S or the number of survivors in the study sample (A) minus the expected (E) number of survivors from TRISS data divided by a statistical (S) variation factor $(Z = S - _{i=1}E^nP_i/_{i=1}E^nP_iQ_i)$[7,26,111]. Survival in the study population better than predicted is indicated by a positive Z-statistic, greater than the upper critical limit of normal standard deviation (α, $p < 0.05$, 1.96), while less than predicted survival is indicated by a negative Z-statistic, less than the lower critical limit (α, $p < 0.05$, –1.96) (Table 9)[7,35,111].

The probability of detecting a difference in survival depends on the size and distribution of the study population combined with the magnitude and direction of the difference from the control population[112]. Significance may be reached by a large difference in a limited population or a small difference in a larger population. Thus, the Z-statistic quantifies group performance, compared to the standard institutional baseline survival.

The W-statistic quantifies the clinical significance of the difference between the study and baseline populations. The W-statistic is equivalent to (A–E)/(N/100), where N represents the sample size[26]. The W-score is expressed as the average increase (positive) or decrease (negative) in number of survivors per 100 patients. Thus, the W-statistic clarifies the clinical significance of the quantitative difference in survival (Table 9). The M-statistic (Table 10) qualifies the 'match' of the study and baseline populations for injury severity. The M-statistic is equivalent to the sum of the fraction of patients falling into subsets of the total group $S_1 + S_2 + S_3 + S_4 + S_5 + S_6$, which is the minimum of similar subsets of the study (g_1–g_n) and baseline (f_1–f_n) populations[101]. If the M-value or the sum of the minimum of subsets is >0.90 (range 0–1.0), then the groups are appropriately matched for statistical and clinical comparison (Table 10).

Another characterization of injury severity is the ASCOT (a severity characterization of trauma) system consisting of four anatomical profile categories for serious (AIS >2) head, brain, spinal cord injuries (A), thorax and front of neck (B), other serious injuries (C) and (D) for all non-serious (AIS 1 or 2) injuries; three coded RTS variables for physiological injury; and age rated by decade (0–4) over 54 years of age[21,113]. This group of 12 845 blunt and 3109 penetrating trauma patients were compared with the TRISS database, and outlyers with extremely poor prognosis, usually cardiac arrest (1: AIS 6/RTS = 0; 2: max AIS <6/RTS = 0; 3: AIS 6/RTS >0), were excluded as 'set asides' from analysis[21,113]. The probability of survival is determined as for

Table 9 Survival statistics: probability of survival of group. Data from references 26, 91, 94, 109–111 and 113

Patient	Survival	P_i	Q_i	P_iQ_i
1	0	0.997	0.003	0.0029
2	0	0.336	0.664	0.2231
3	1	0.778	0.222	0.1727
4	1	0.995	0.005	0.0049
5	1	0.865	0.135	0.1167
6	0	0.455	0.545	0.2479
7	1	0.991	0.009	0.0089
8	0	0.686	0.314	0.2154
9	0	0.547	0.453	0.2477
10	1	0.771	0.229	0.1765
Total	5	7.421	2.579	1.4167

$$Z = \frac{S - {}_{i=1}E^nP_i}{\sqrt{{}^nE_{i=1}\,P_iQ_i}} = \frac{S - E\,P_i}{E\,P_iQ_i}$$

where Z-statistic is difference in survival between experimental and baseline populations; ($Z < -1.96$, decreased survival; $Z > 1.96$, increased survival); patient (i) = 0 death, 1 survivor; P_i is the probability of survival; $Q_i = 1 - P_i$ is the probability of death; and S is total survivors.

Example:
$$Z = \frac{5 - 7.421}{1.4167} = \frac{-2.421}{1.1902} = -2.034$$

Survival rate of study population is worse, compared to control population

$$W = \frac{A - E}{N/100}$$

where W-statistic is clinical significance of Z-statistic difference: average increase or decrease in survivors per 100 patients (positive, increased survival; negative, decreased survival); A is actual; E is expected; and N is sample size.

Example:
$$W = \frac{5 - 7.421}{10/100} = -24.21 \text{ per } 100$$

Significant decrease in survival is exacerbated with small sample size.

Table 10 Survival statistics: probability of survival of group. Data from references 26, 91, 94, 101, 111 and 113

P_s	Study (g)	Baseline (f)	Minimum
0.96–1.00	0.300	0.500	0.300
0.91–0.95	0.000	0.100	0.000
0.76–0.90	0.200	0.100	0.100
0.51–0.75	0.300	0.100	0.100
0.26–0.50	0.200	0.100	0.100
0.00–0.25	0.000	0.100	0.000
Total			0.6

$$M = S_1 + S_2 + S_3 + S_4 + S_5 + S_6$$

where M-statistic is adequacy of match between study and baseline populations, sum of minimum subset values S.

Example: patient range:
$$M = 0.300 + 0.000 + 0.100 + 0.100 + 0.100 + 0.000 = 0.6$$

Sample and baseline populations were significantly different and match was poor (< 0.88)

TRISS analysis: $P_s = 1/1 + e^{-K}$, where $K = K_1 + K_2G + K_3S + K_4R + K_5A + K_6B + K_7C + K_8(age)$[21,113]. Thus, this method uses the injury severity expressed as the square root of the sum of the AIS squares for regions A, B and C, combined with the coded RTS values (G, S and R) and age (Table 11)[21,113].

The advantages of this system include a separate outcome for blunt or penetrating trauma patients, a consideration of all anatomical injury instead of that for only the most severely injured regions and an improvement in sensitivity (from 81.6 to 86.1%), compared to TRISS methodology[21].

The ability to analyze patients' outcome according to objective indices that have the capacity to be modified as the database changes is desirable, and sample calculations are included (Tables 8–11). Trauma audit that relies on retrospective clinical peer review may overestimate preventable deaths in the critically ill, while statistical methods often overestimate survivability in those with less severe (ISS 9–24) injury[114]. Review of trauma complications in a 4744-patient sample suggests that

Table 11 Survival statistics: probability of survival of individual. Data from references 21 and 113

Variable	Description/ injury	AIS severity	ISS body region	ASCOT database coefficients Blunt	Penetrating
Constant				−1.1570	−1.1350
G	Glasgow coma score (GCS)			0.7705	1.0626
S	systolic blood pressure (SBP)			0.6583	0.3638
R	respiratory rate (RR)			0.2810	0.3332
A	head/brain	3–5	1	−0.3002	−0.3702
	spinal cord	3–5	1, 3, 4		
B	thoracic	3–5	3	−0.1962	−0.2053
	front of neck	3–5	1		
C	abdomen/pelvis	3–5	4	−0.2086	−0.3188
	spine without cord	3	1, 3, 4		
	pelvic fracture	4–5	5		
	crush above knee	4–5	5		
	amputation above knee	4–5	5		
	popliteal artery	4	5		
	face	1–4	2		
D	all others	1–2	1–6		
Age	0, 0–54 years; 1, 55–64 years; 2, 65–74 years; 3, 75–84 years; 4, ≥ 85 years			−0.6355	0.8365

$$P_s = \frac{1}{1 + e^{-K}}$$

where P_s is probability of survival, and $K = K_1 + K_2G + K_3S + K_4R + K_5A + K_6B + K_7C + K_8(\text{age})$ (all non-serious injury excluded: category D, AIS 1–2).

Table 11 Continued

Table 11 *Continued*

Variable	Description/ injury	AIS severity	ISS body region	ASCOT database coefficients	
				Blunt	Penetrating

Example: A 63-year-old male presents with fall from height with GCS (8), SBP (70 mmHg) and RR = 40. Injuries include a basilar skull fracture (AIS 3), bilateral hemothorax (AIS 4) and minor L1 compression fracture (AIS 2) with an ISS of 29:

$$K = (-1.1570) + 0.7705(2) + 0.6583(2) + 0.2810(3) + [-0.3002(3)] + [-0.1962(4)] + [-0.2086(0)] + [-0.6355(1)]$$
$$= (-1.1570) + (1.5410) + (1.3166) + (0.8430) + (-0.9006) + (-0.7848) + (0) + (-0.6355)$$
$$= 0.2227$$

$$P_s = \frac{1}{1 + 2.718\,282^{-0.2227}}$$
$$= 0.5554$$

Probability of survival is 55.5%

AIS, abbreviated injury scale; ISS, injury severity scale; ASCOT, a severity characterization of trauma

759 (16%) of patients had provider-related complications with 175 (23%) felt to be unjustified[115]. There were 16 patterns of recurrent process of care errors, including delay in trauma team activation, delay in diagnosis or surgery, error in technique and/or error in judgement[115].

REHABILITATION

The long-term (5-year) outcome based predominantly on Tiret and colleagues' evaluation[116] of 8940 and Frutiger and co-workers' evaluation[117] of 223 patients after rehabilitation for acute traumatic injury is favorable, with slight disability in most (87%) patients, followed by severe dysfunction in 10% and a persistent vegetative state in 3% (Table 12)[118]. The patients' ability to recover cognitive function is often underestimated by health-care professionals, with over 77% of patients in these studies returning to their baseline mental status.

Table 12 Disability after traumatic injury. Data from references 116–118

| | Glasgow Outcome Score | Incidence (%) | |
		Range	Cumulative
Mortality		4–51	26
Disability			
Slight	4, 5	80–90	87
Severe	2, 3	9–11	10
Persistent vegetative state	1	0–8	3
Mental status			
Normal			77
Dementia			23

The most important issue to address is subsequent quality of life. Although Hackl and associates' evaluation[119] of 106 patients with minor head injury showed that all were able to return to activities of daily living level, only 50% returned to their normal social structure and 29% remained unemployed. The investigation of Pauser and colleagues[120] revealed that as many as 73% of 182 head injury patients have intermittent moderate levels of dysfunction and 27% severe dysfunction, specifically suicidal ideation (39%) and drug dependence (35%). The presentation of GCS admission scores and persistent post-trauma amnesia were often indicators for poor future recovery in Stambrook and co-workers' evaluation[121] of severely injured patients. Disappointingly, only half of these patients were able to return to active employment after significant head injury[121].

Neuropsychiatric testing by Mayes and associates[122] of a 34-patient head trauma group revealed that those with the highest preinjury intelligence quotients (IQs) had the greatest post-traumatic deficit. One method of classifying neuropsychiatric deficits is the Halstead–Reitan impairment index, which correlates with GCS, ISS and employment status[123,124]. Good recovery was associated with a healthy premorbid condition, absence of psychiatric dysfunction, lack of persistent physical disability and stable employment, while spinal fracture, pupillary dysfunction and intracranial pressure elevation were associated with impaired neurophysiological testing, in Gensemer and colleagues' evaluation[123] of 65 head-injured patients.

CONCLUSION

Outcome is determined in part by a patient's age and medical condition, the mechanism of trauma, the presence of head injury or visceral trauma and the quality of the rehabilitation. The most significant adverse prognostic predictor is the presence of significant persistent head injury, but this does not eliminate the likelihood of a positive outcome completely. Physicians often underestimate patients' ability to recover. However, each successive day of persistent coma or organ system dysfunction makes complete recovery less likely. Aggressive intensive care intervention is crucial to minimize secondary post-traumatic insult due to organ system dysfunction caused by oxygen delivery and consumption imbalance.

REFERENCES

1. Uzych L. Trauma care systems. *Am J Emerg Med* 1990;8:71–5
2. Potter D, Goldstein G, Fung SC, *et al.* A controlled trial of prehospital advanced life support in trauma. *Ann Emerg Med* 1988;17:582–8
3. Schwartz RJ, Jacobs LM, Yaezel D. Impact of pre-trauma center care on length of stay and hospital charges. *J Trauma* 1989;29:1611–15
4. Schmidt U, Frame SB, Nerlich L, *et al.* On-scene helicopter transport of patients with multiple injuries – comparison of a German and an American system. *J Trauma* 1992;33:548–53
5. West JG, Williams MJ, Trunkey DD, *et al.* Trauma systems current status – future challenges. *J Am Med Assoc* 1988;259:3597
6. American College of Surgeons. *Hospital and prehospital resources for optimal care of the injured patient.* ACS, Chicago, 1987
7. American College of Surgeons. *Resources for optimal care of the injured patient.* ACS, Chicago, 1993:1–4
8. Baker CC, Degutis LC, DeSantis J, *et al.* Impact of a trauma service on trauma care in a university hospital. *Am J Surg* 1985;149:453–8
9. Clemmer TP, Orme JF Jr, Thomas FO, *et al.* Outcome of critically injured patients treated at level I trauma centers versus full-service community hospitals. *Crit Care Med* 1985;13:861–3
10. Smith JS Jr, Martin LF, Young WW, *et al.* Do trauma centers improve outcome over non-trauma centers: the evaluation of regional trauma care using discharge abstract data and patient management categories. *J Trauma* 1990;30:1533–8

11. Mullins RJ, Veum-Stone J, Helfand M, *et al.* Outcome of hospitalized injured patients after institution of a trauma system in an urban area. *J Am Med Assoc* 1994;271:1919–24

12. Waddell TK, Kalman PG, Goodman SJL, *et al.* Is outcome worse in a small volume Canadian trauma centre? *J Trauma* 1991;31:958–61

13. Karsteadt LL, Larsen CL, Farmer PD. Analysis of a rural trauma program using the TRISS methodology: a three-year retrospective study. *J Trauma* 1994;36:395–400

14. Norwood S, Myers MB. Outcomes following injury in a predominantly rural-population-based trauma center. *Arch Surg* 1994;129: 800–5

15. Shackford SR, Mackersie RC, Hoyt DB, *et al.* Impact of a trauma system on outcome of severely injured patients. *Arch Surg* 1987;122:523–7

16. Weiland DE, Malone JM, Krebs R, *et al.* Trauma malpractice claims related to trauma level designation. *Am J Surg* 1989;158:553–6

17. Thompson CT, Bickell WH, Siemens RA, *et al.* Community hospital level II trauma center outcome. *J Trauma* 1992;32:336–41

18. Barone JE, Ryan MC, Cayten CG, *et al.* Is 24-hour operating room staff absolutely necessary for level II trauma center designation? *J Trauma* 1993;34:878–82

19. Morris JA, MacKenzie EJ, Edelstein SL. The effect of preexisting conditions on mortality in trauma patients. *J Am Med Assoc* 1990;263: 1942–6

20. Morris JA Jr, MacKenzie EJ, Damiano AM, *et al.* Mortality in trauma patients: the interaction between host factors and severity. *Crit Care Med* 1990;30:1476–82

21. Sacco WJ, Copes WS, Bain LW Jr, *et al.* Effect of preinjury illness on trauma patient survival outcome. *J Trauma* 1993;35:538–42

22. Pollack MM, Alexander SR, Clarke N, *et al.* Improved outcomes from tertiary center pediatric intensive care: a statewide comparison of tertiary and nontertiary care facilities. *Crit Care Med* 1991;19:150–9

23. Nakayama DK, Copes WS, Sacco WJ. The effect of patient age upon survival in pediatric trauma. *J Trauma* 1991;31:1521–6

24. Tepas JJ 3rd, Mollitt DL, Talbert JL, *et al.* The pediatric trauma score as a predictor of injury severity in the injured child. *J Pediatr Surg* 1987; 22:14–18

25. Knudson MM, Shagoury C, Lewis FR. Can adult trauma surgeons care for injured children? *J Trauma* 1992;32:729–37

26. Champion HR, Copes WS, Sacco WJ, *et al.* The major trauma outcome study: establishing national norms for trauma care. *J Trauma* 1990;30: 1356–65

27. Bensard DD, McIntyre RC Jr, Moore EE, *et al*. A critical analysis of acutely injured children managed in an adult level I trauma center. *J Pediatr Surg* 1994;29:8–11

28. Smith DP, Enderson BL, Maull KI. Trauma in the elderly. Determinants of outcome. *South Med J* 1990;83:171–7

29. van Aalst JA, Morris JA Jr, Yates HK, *et al*. Severely injured geriatric patients return to independent living: a study of factors influencing function and independence. *J Trauma* 1991;31:1096–101

30. DeMaria EJ, Kenney PR, Merriam MA, *et al*. Aggressive trauma care benefits the elderly. *J Trauma* 1987;27:1200–6

31. Finelli FC, Jonsson J, Champion HR, *et al*. A case control study for major trauma in geriatric patients. *J Trauma* 1989;29:541–8

32. Grenrot C, Hakansson N, Hakansson S. Intensive care of the elderly – a retrospective study. *Acta Anaesthesiol Scand* 1986;30:703–8

33. Wilson B, Vizor A, Bryant T. Predicting severity of cognitive impairment after severe head injury. *Brain Inj* 1991;5:189–97

34. Thomsen IV. Do young patients have worse outcomes after severe blunt head trauma? *Brain Inj* 1989;3:157–62

35. Rubli E, Bussard S, Frei E, *et al*. Plasma fibronectin and associated variables in surgical intensive care patients. *Ann Surg* 1983;197: 310–17

36. Christou NV, Tellado JM. *In vitro* polymorphonuclear neutrophil function in surgical patients does not correlate with anergy but with 'activating' processes such as sepsis or trauma. *Surgery* 1989;106:718–24

37. Wolmann A, Kress HG. The prognostic value of the delayed cutaneous immune reaction following multiple trauma in comparison with other clinical parameters. *Anaesthetist* 1991;40:276–81

38. Visser JJ, Meyer S, deJong D. Phytohemagglutinin skin testing in critically ill surgical patients. *Acute Care* 1986;12:52–7

39. Kabisch S, Gemar K, Krumholz W, *et al*. Lymphocyte subpopulations in patients at risk of sepsis in a surgical intensive care unit. *Anaesthetist* 1990;39:439–44

40. Fiennes AG, Gudgeion AM, Jehanli A, *et al*. Released phospholipase A2 activation peptides in the rapid early prediction of trauma outcome: a preliminary report. *Injury* 1991;22:219–22

41. Sturaitis M, McCallum D, Sutherland G, *et al*. Lack of significant long-term sequelae following traumatic myocardial contusion. *Arch Intern Med* 1986;146:1765–9

42. Rady MY, Edwards JD, Nightingale P. Early cardiorespiratory findings after severe blunt thoracic trauma and their relation to outcome. *Br J Surg* 1992;79:65–8

43. Scalea TM, Simon HM, Duncan AO, *et al.* Geriatric blunt multiple trauma: improved survival with early invasive monitoring. *J Trauma* 1990;30:129–35

44. Lee RB, Morris JA, Parker RS. Presence of three or more rib fractures as an indicator of need for interhospital transfer. *J Trauma* 1989;29:795–9

45. Fussle R, Biscoping J, Zeiler D, *et al.* Microbiological care of ventilated intensive care patients. Feasibility of diagnosis and therapy of pulmonary infection. *Anaesthetist* 1991;40:491–6

46. Corwin HL, Sprague SM, DeLaria GA, *et al.* Acute renal failure associated with cardiac operations. A case–control study. *J Thoracic Cardiovasc Surg* 1989;98:1107–12

47. Mukau L, Latimer RG. Acute hemodialysis in the surgical intensive care unit. *Am Surg* 1988;54:548–52

48. Wheeler DC, Feehally J, Walls J. High risk acute renal failure. *Q J Med* 1986;61:977–84

49. Foco A, Giordano A, Passarelli E, *et al.* Postoperative treatment of liver injuries in the surgical intensive care unit. *Minerva Med* 1981;72:17–20

50. Cornwell EE, Rodriguez A, Mirvis SE, *et al.* Acute acalculous cholecystitis in critically injured patients. Preoperative diagnostic imaging. *Ann Surg* 1989;210:52–5

51. Wardrope J, Cross SF, Fothergill DJ. One year's experience of major trauma outcome study methodology. *Br Med J* 1990;301:156–9

52. Enderson BL, Reath DB, Meadors J, *et al.* The tertiary trauma survey: a prospective study of missed injury. *J Trauma* 1990;30:666–70

53. Poole GV, Ward EF, Muakkassa FF. Pelvic fracture from major blunt trauma. Outcome is determined by associated injuries. *Ann Surg* 1991; 213:532–8

54. Manship L, McMillin RD, Brown JJ. The influence of sepsis and multisystem organ failure on mortality in the surgical intensive care unit. *Am Surg* 1984;50:94–101

55. Levi L, Borovich B, Guilburd JN, *et al.* Wartime neurosurgical experience in Lebanon, 1982–85. II: Closed craniocerebral injuries. *Isr J Med Sci* 1990;26:555–8

56. Grewal M, Sutcliffe AJ. Early prediction of outcome following head injury in children: an assessment of the value of Glasgow coma scale score trend and abnormal plantar and pupillary light reflexes. *J Pediatr Surg* 1991;26:1161–3

57. Waxman K, Sundine MJ, Young RF. Is early prediction of outcome in severe head injury possible? *Arch Surg* 1991;126:1237–41

58. Marshall LF, Gautille T, Klauber MR, *et al.* The outcome of severe closed head injury. *J Neurosurg* 1991;75:S28–36

59. Meier U, Knopf W, Klotzer R, *et al.* Postoperative results following severe craniocerebral trauma. *Zentralbl Chir* 1991;116:845–54

60. Bricolo A, Turazzi S, Feriotti G. Prolonged posttraumatic unconsciousness: therapeutic assets and liabilities. *J Neurosurg* 1980;52:625–34

61. Andrews BT, Chiles BW 3rd, Olsen WL, *et al.* The effect of intracerebral hematoma location on the risk of brain-stem compression and on clinical outcome. *J Neurosurg* 1988;69:518–22

62. Marshall LF, Marshall SB, Klauber MR, *et al.* A new classification of head injury based on computerized tomography. *J Neurosurg* 1991;75: S14–20

63. Warme PE, Bergstrom R, Persson L. Neurosurgical intensive care improves outcome after severe head injury. *Acta Neurochir* 1991;110: 57–64

64. Miller JD, Becker DP, Ward JD, *et al.* Significance of intracranial hypertension in severe head injury. *J Neurosurg* 1977;47:503–16

65. Marmarou A, Anderson RL, Ward JD, *et al.* NINDS traumatic coma data bank: intracranial pressure monitoring methodology. *J Neurosurg* 1991;75:S21–7

66. Stocchetti N, Paparella, Serioli T, *et al.* Cerebral perfusion pressure in endocranial hypertension in comatose head-injured patients. *Minerva Anestesiol* 1990;56:27–32

67. Miller JD, Jones PA, Dearden NM, *et al.* Progress in the management of head injury. *Br J Surg* 1992;79:60–4

68. Vollmer DG, Torner JC, Jane JA, *et al.* Age and outcome following traumatic coma: why do older patients fare worse? *J Neurosurg* 1991;75: S37–49

69. Shackford SR, Mackersie RC, Davis JW, *et al.* Epidemiology and pathology of traumatic deaths occurring at a level I trauma center in a regionalized system: the importance of secondary brain injury. *J Trauma* 1989;29:1392–7

70. Crawford C. Social problems after severe head injury. *NZ Med J* 1983;96:972–4

71. Foulkes MA, Eisenberg HM, Jane JA, *et al.* The traumatic coma data bank: design, methods and baseline characteristics. *J Neurosurg* 1991;75:S8–13

72. Levin HS, Saydjari C, Eisenberg HM, *et al.* Vegetative state after closed-head injury. A traumatic coma data bank report. *Arch Neurol* 1991;48:580–5

73. Glinz W, Ruckert R. Cost and benefit of intensive care of seriously injured patients. *Schweiz Med Wochenschr* 1988;118:643–8

74. DeVivo MJ, Kartus PL, Stover SL, *et al.* Cause of death for patients with spinal cord injuries. *Arch Intern Med* 1989;149:1761–6

75. Bracken MB, Shepard MJ, Collins WF, *et al.* A randomized, controlled trial of methylprednisolone or naloxone in the treatment of acute spinal-cord injury. *N Engl J Med* 1990;322:1405–11
76. Geisler FH, Dorsey FC, Coleman WP. Recovery of motor function after spinal-cord injury – a randomized, placebo-controlled trial with GM-1 ganglioside. *N Engl J Med* 1991;324:1829–38
77. Frankel HL, Hyslop HG, Melzak HJ, *et al.* The value of postural reduction in the initial management of closed injuries of the spine with paraplegia and tetraplegia. *Paraplegia* 1969;7:179–92
78. American Spinal Injury Association. *Standards for neurological classification of spinal injury patients.* American Spinal Injury Association, Chicago, 1984
79. Gerhart KA. Spinal cord injury outcomes in a population-based sample. *J Trauma* 1991;31:1529–35
80. Heinemann AW, Yarkony GM, Roth EJ, *et al.* Functional outcome following spinal cord injury. *Arch Neurol* 1989;46:1098–102
81. Knaus WA, Draper EA, Wagner DP, *et al.* Prognosis in acute organ-system failure. *Ann Surg* 1985;202:685–93
82. Crump JM, Duncan DA, Wears R. Analysis of multiple organ system failure in trauma and nontrauma patients. *Am Surg* 1988;54:702–8
83. Darling GE, Duff JH, Mustard RA, *et al.* Multiorgan failure in critically ill patients. *Can J Surg* 1988;31:172–6
84. Knaus WA, Wagner DP, Draper EA. Relationship between acute physiologic derangement and risk of death. *J Chronic Dis* 1985;38:295–300
85. Teasdale G, Jennett B. Assessment of coma and impaired consciousness: a practical scale. *Lancet* 1974;2:81–3
86. Champion HR, Sacco WJ, Carnazzo AJ, *et al.* Trauma score. *Crit Care Med* 1981;9:672–6
87. Champion HR, Sacco WJ, Copes WS, *et al.* A revision of the trauma score. *J Trauma* 1989;29:623–9
88. Kaufmann CR, Maier RV, Rivara FP, *et al.* Evaluation of the pediatric trauma score. *J Am Med Assoc* 1990;263:69–72
89. Gormican SP. CRAMS scale: field triage of trauma victims. *Ann Emerg Med* 1982;11:132–5
90. Committee on Medical Aspects of Automotive Safety. Rating the severity of tissue damage. *J Am Med Assoc* 1971;215:277–80
91. Baker SP, O'Neill B, Haddon W Jr, *et al.* The injury severity score: a method for describing patients with multiple injuries and evaluating emergency care. *J Trauma* 1974;14:187–96
92. Baker SP, O'Neil B. The injury severity score. An update. *J Trauma* 1976;16:882–5
93. Civil ID, Schwab CW. The abbreviated injury scale, 1985 revision: a condensed chart for clinical use. *J Trauma* 1988;26:87–90

94. American Association for Automotive Medicine. *The abbreviated injury scale, 1985 revision*. American Association for Automotive Medicine, Des Plines, IL, 1985

95. Kramer CF, Barancik JI, Thode HC Jr. Improving the sensitivity and specificity of the abbreviated injury scale coding system. *Public Health Rep* 1990;105:334–40

96. MacKenzie EJ, Shapiro S, Eastham JN. The abbreviated injury scale and injury severity score. *Med Care* 1985;23:823–35

97. Committee on Medical Aspects of Automotive Safety. Rating the severity of tissue damage. *J Am Med Assoc* 1972;220:717–20

98. Jennett B, Bond M. Assessment of outcome after severe brain damage: a practical scale. *Lancet* 1975;1:480–5

99. Cullen DJ, Civetta JM, Briggs BA, *et al.* Therapeutic intervention scoring system: a method for quantitative comparison of patient care. *Crit Care Med* 1974;2:57–60

100. Keene AR, Cullen DJ. Therapeutic intervention scoring system: update 1983. *Crit Care Med* 1983;11:1–3

101. Boyd CR, Tolson MA, Copes WS. Evaluating trauma care: the TRISS method. *J Trauma* 1987;27:370–8

102. Knaus WA, Zimmerman JE, Wagner DP, *et al.* APACHE – acute physiology and chronic health evaluation: a physiologically based classification system. *Crit Care Med* 1981;9:591–7

103. Knaus WA, Draper EA, Wagner DP, *et al.* APACHE II: a severity of disease classification system. *Crit Care Med* 1985;13:818–29

104. Knaus WA, Wagner DP, Draper EA, *et al.* The APACHE III prognostic system risk prediction of hospital mortality for critically ill hospitalized adults. *Chest* 1991;100:1619–36

105. Lemeshow S, Teres D, Pastides H, *et al.* A method for predicting survival and mortality of ICU patients using objectively derived weights. *Crit Care Med* 1985;13:519–25

106. Zimmerman JE, Knaus WA, Judson JA, *et al.* Patient selection for intensive care: a comparison of New Zealand and United States hospitals. *Crit Care Med* 1988;16:318–26

107. Kaukinen L, Pasanen M, Kaukinen S. Outcome and risk factors in severely traumatized patients. *Ann Chir Gynaecol* 1984;73:261–7

108. Schiowitz MF. Patient throughput and mortality rate in a trauma service. *Br J Surg* 1990;77:497–8

109. Beeko A, Ramsen M, Baz OA, *et al.* Interventions in polytrauma in the kingdom of Saudi Arabia. A study of 310 polytraumatized patients. *Neurosurg Rev* 1989;12:S17–21

110. Champion HR, Sacco WJ, Hunt TK. Trauma severity scoring to predict mortality. *World J Surg* 1983;7:4–11

111. Flora JD Jr. A method for comparing survival of burn patients to a standard survival curve. *J Trauma* 1978;18:701–5

112. Cottington EM, Shufflebarger CM, Townsend R. The power of the Z statistic: implications for trauma research and quality assurance review. *J Trauma* 1989;29:1500–9

113. Champion HR, Copes WS, Sacco WJ, *et al.* A new characterization of injury severity. *J Trauma* 1990;30:539–45

114. Yates DW, Woodford M, Hollis S, *et al.* Trauma audit: clinical judgement or statistical analysis? *Ann R Coll Surg Engl* 1993;75:321–4

115. Hoyt DV, Hollingsworth-Fridlund P, Winchell RJ, *et al.* Analysis of recurrent process errors leading to provider-related complications in an organized trauma service: directions for care improvement. *J Trauma* 1994;36:377–84

116. Tiret L, Hausherr E, Thicoipe M, *et al.* The epidemiology of head trauma in Aquitatine, 1986: a community-based study of hospital admissions and deaths. *Int J Epidemiol* 1990;19:133–40

117. Frutiger A, Ryf C, Bilat C, *et al.* Five years' follow-up of severely injured ICU patients. *J Trauma* 1991;31:1216–25

118. Oder W, Goldenberg G, Podreka I, *et al.* HM–PAO–SPECT in persistent vegetative state after head injury: prognostic indicator of the likelihood of recovery? *Intens Care Med* 1991;17:149–53

119. Hackl JM, Benzer A, Putz G, *et al.* How much reintegration can be achieved in patients after severe craniocerebral injury? *Anaesthetist* 1986;35:171–6

120. Pauser G, Benzer H, Bunzel B, *et al.* Intensive medicine – and what follows? Psychosocial follow-up study of former intensive care patients [in German]. *Anaesthetist* 1984;33:189–95

121. Stambrook M, Moore AD, Peters LC, *et al.* Effects of mild, moderate and severe closed head injury on long-term vocational status. *Brain Inj* 1990;492:183–90

122. Mayes SD, Pelco LE, Campbell CJ. Relationships among pre- and post-injury intelligence, length of coma and age in individuals with severe closed-head injuries. *Brain Inj* 1989;3:301–13

123. Gensemer IB, McMurry FG, Walker JC, *et al.* Behavioral consequences of trauma. *J Trauma* 1988;28:44–9

124. Reitan RM. *The Halstead–Reitan Neurophysiological Test Battery: Theory and Clinical Interpretation.* Tucson, AZ: Neuropsychology Press, 1985

Index